Praise for *The Cat's Got Nothing on Me*

"Conrad 'Chickie' Boilard leaves us his insightful views on how to cope with the problems of life. Everything from the title to the end of the book is filled with his special humor and warmth that was contagious to all those around him. It was an honor to have been able to serve him as his physician. A pleasant surprise that he held me in the esteem he did and a great sense of satisfaction to have helped keep him close to those he loved the most. In today's world of disposable relationships it is enlightening to read a book about a man who drew strength from his family and friends to help him in the toughest of times. Truly, Chick, you left us all the best of legacies — humor, perseverance, and loyalty to family and friends. All of us who knew and met you were truly blessed."

—David F. Fernandez, M.D. FACP
Chick's physician

"Chick's stories of survival and endless optimism in the face of life-threatening illnesses and accidents bring a chuckle and a smile. This simple story of a not-so-simple life will encourage anyone facing life's trials and tribulations."

—Teresa Rafferty, Ph.D.
Family Therapist

"If you like smiles, a good laugh, some encouragement, and a great example of "get up, brush yourself off, and start all over again," then Chick's story is for you. Always a gentlemen, always ready with a good story, and always an encourager, this book tells you how he became what he was. Nearly drowning, kidney stones, and cancer will either take you down or build you up. Chick became stronger and gives us words of wisdom, all packed with humor, to help us do the same. Although he will be terribly missed, the great memories never leave."

—Charles Reinersten, DMD
Chick's dentist in Florida

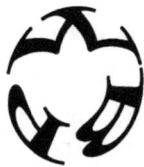

Wandering Brothers
Publishing, CO

THE CAT'S GOT NOTHING ON ME

FIRST PRINTING: APRIL 2006

PUBLISHED BY WANDERING BROTHERS PUBLISHING
419 PLATEAU DRIVE,
FLORISSANT, CO 80816
WWW.WANDERINGBROTHERS.COM

Dedicated to:

My wife, Marie, who made it all possible

My doctors, with respect and admiration

My family, with gratitude

My extended family and friends, with love

The Cat's Got Nothing on Me

How I Lived More Than Nine Lives

By Conrad Boilard
as told to Sam Costello

Introduction

My name is Conrad "Chickie" Boilard and I am a survivor. I have survived two heart attacks, three kinds of cancer, almost drowning, a near plane-crash, being run over by a truck, heart bypass surgery, and the rigors of war. You could say that I've lived more lives than a cat.

When I tell people my stories of survival they seem amazed. People suffering from chronic or life-threatening illnesses tell me they find hope in my stories. More than once someone has told me that I ought to write my stories down. Now I have.

The stories that follow are meant to guide you, to inspire you. They're not a set of rules or a path you can follow step by step. That would be preaching and I don't preach. You need to understand your story, your history, and find your own pockets of strength, just as I've found mine. My hope is that these stories will help you in your search for survival, strength, and wisdom.

As I started work on this book, I began to wonder where I got my strength of spirit. Thinking back on it, I realized that everything that got me through in later life – humor, hard work, laughter, love – came from my parents and my brothers and sister. My family, I realized, is a major part of how I became who I am.

So my story begins with them.

Chapter 1
The Foundation of My Strength

I was born on August 5, 1924, in Ludlow, Massachusetts, to Adelard and Lillian Boilard. Dad worked for the Tebaldi Concrete Block Company in Indian Orchard, Massachusetts, a town about a mile and a half from Ludlow and nine miles from Springfield. We lived in a home across the street from the plant.

I was the fourth child – and the third son - in the family. Coming before me was Edward, who was 6 years older than me, then our one sister, Lillian, four years older than me, and William, two years older than me. Six years after I was born came our youngest brother, Bobby.

Though my parents named me Conrad, those who know me have called me "Chickie" (and later "Chick") almost all my life. I got the name from my dad's brother Fred. When I was five or six years old, Fred took me – dressed in a little sailor suit – to visit some relatives on the Connecticut coast. While visiting, we went to a chicken coop. I loved running around with the birds and chasing them. After I did that and a few people saw me, everyone started to call "chick, chick, chick" after me, making the noise a chicken would make.

Chapter 1: The Foundation of My Strength

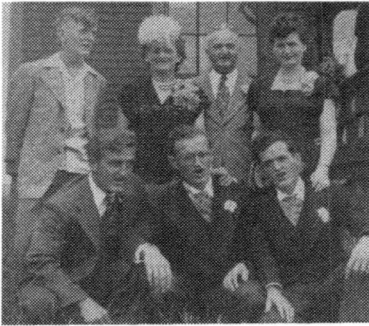

My family and me
(I'm at the bottom right).

It progressed from there. My parents started calling me "Chick" or "Chickie" and then my brothers and sister picked it up and it's been my nickname ever since.

My aunt, Uncle Fred and dad's sister, didn't like the nickname. She tried for a more traditional nickname instead, calling me "Connie," short for Conrad. I didn't like that name, though, because to me Connie was a girl's name. It didn't stick.

Just a few years after I was born, the country entered the Great Depression (I'm pretty sure the two events were unrelated) and stayed in it until my teens. The Depression hit Springfield pretty hard and dad worked equally hard to make a living for us. His days were long - sometimes six in the morning until after five at night - for around $19 a week. For that pay, dad also would stoke the fires of coal furnaces in the neighborhood, a job he'd sometimes bring me and Billy with him on. Nineteen dollars a week wasn't a lot, but we were able to get by and it was more than a lot of other people had. At least dad had work, and his pay also included the rent on the house from Tebaldi. We didn't have much, but we didn't want for much, either.

Even though we didn't have a lot of money, we found ways to entertain ourselves for free. For instance, my relatives who lived in the area would often come over to the house at night to play music. It was uncles and cousins who would come, bringing their instruments and gathering around the piano. They'd play as a band, singing traditional songs like "Home on the Range" and having a great old time. Us kids were too young to join in, but we watched and listened and we loved it.

When we were growing up, my dad was the master of the house. Of course, this isn't how things are today, but they were different back then. The mother stayed home, cooked, cleaned, and tended to the kids. The father went to work and earned the money. I still think this is the way it should be, even though my daughters get mad whenever I say it.

Still, just because dad was the boss at home didn't stop us from having fun with him. My dad had a wonderful sense of humor throughout his 86 years. His humor was sometimes subtle and dry, other times outrageous. Not every father was able to find humor and fun during the Depression, but he did. My dad blessed all his children with a healthy sense of humor.

But dad had a serious side, too. Every night after dinner, he would go upstairs to study his Hamilton Business course. His dream was to someday own his own business and so he took it on himself to learn what he needed to know about running one. Our orders from mom were not to disturb him while he studied. Eventually he finished his course and realized his dream, founding and owning his own concrete and building supply business in 1936. He called the new company A. Boilard Sons.

When dad started that business, he did it on trust. When he decided to set out on his own, a salesman he knew from his previous job offered his trust and gave him good terms on his first order so he could get a solid start. A neighbor offered him free use of space at his business so dad could store that first order until he got established.

People made these offers because they knew my dad and trusted him. Trust was everything to these people and it was crucial to my dad's success. If these people hadn't known him and hadn't taken a chance on him, he probably couldn't have gotten the business off the ground.

Trust is important and so is good luck. My dad once ordered four sets of boxes of shingles from a salesman, sight unseen. My dad thought each set was going to hold a small number of boxes and boy was he surprised when they showed up with two or three times more boxes on each one than he expected! He didn't know how he was going to sell them all and was worried for the health of his company.

Then, just a day or two after the shingles were delivered, the Hurricane of 1938 struck Springfield.

For those of you who don't remember, the Hurricane of 1938 was a pretty big deal. After it hit, they counted and found that it had killed 600 people, injured 3,500, and destroyed over 7,500 buildings around New York and New England. The worst-hit places were on the water, of course, like Long Island and the Rhode Island coast. Providence, Rhode Island, got flooded with 14 feet of water and some people were stranded inside downtown buildings!

Even as far inland as where we were, the storm was pretty tough. We had hurricane-type winds – and you know what those do to roofs!

What they do to shingles, they almost did to me, too. The day the hurricane came, I hadn't heard much about it – this was long before 24-hour news or the Internet, remember. So, I was in the lumberyard and one of dad's workers drove up in a truck. He had a load to deliver and asked me if I wanted to come with him. I said yes and hopped in.

We drove down State St. in Ludlow and the wind was blowing hard, so hard that the trees lining it were bent down to the ground. That's when I knew something unusual was happening, though I still didn't know what it was.

The wind was picking up something fierce and as we drove down the street I saw a man sitting in his car reading the newspaper. All of a sudden, a tree blew over in front of him and fell into his car, crushing its hood. Further down the street, all of the glass had been blown out of the windows of the drugstore and there was a man inside eating an ice cream!

It turned out that the delivery my dad's employee was making was a load of sand bags to dam up the Connecticut River to prevent it from overflowing. The storm got too bad, though, and we had to turn around for our safety. That delivery was never made.

The winds that blew so hard as to break glass and knock down trees also destroyed a lot of roofs in the area. Shingles were torn off and a lot of houses were bare on the top.

The next day, we had dozens of people looking to get new shingles for their houses. My sister Lillian set up a cash box on a barrel head and we sold out of the whole order of shingles right away and dad made a good profit. Our shingles were brown while those on many people's roofs were black, so for years throughout Springfield you could see houses with mixed brown and black shingles. Those were ours!

Without that hurricane, dad's business might not have made it. So having the right circumstances has always been important to me. Even more than that, having God operating in your life is important.

But we didn't just rely on God or circumstance. We relied on our hands and backs and sweat, too. We worked hard. Boy, did we work hard! All the kids worked at my dad's business. Lillian was his secretary from the moment he opened the company and the rest of us worked moving bags of concrete, loading and unloading shipments. At just the age of 12, I helped unload the first order of cement delivered to my dad.

We lived close together, had fun together, and worked hard together. I was always close with my brothers and sister, especially Billy and Edward.

Billy and I were like partners in crime. We'd have fun together and get into trouble together. We used to tease Lillian a lot, as brothers do to their sisters. We always used to open her Christmas presents before Christmas morning came. This made her cry, but it didn't stop us.

To scare Lillian, we once took a bathrobe and tied a rope around its neck. We then threw the whole bundle over a railing and let it hang down over the stairs so that it looked like a hanged body. This scared Lillian badly. We loved it.

Luckily as we grew older and more mature, we developed the good, close relationships that we have now.

As much trouble as Billy and I got in, I got advice to balance it out from Edward. He was my priest, my lawyer, my banker, my councilor. I went to him with everything, all my questions, all my troubles, except for ones about sex.

When we weren't in school, we worked from sun up to sun down at the business. When we got old enough, we'd knock off work and head to town for a cold beer — but always just one.

To make the work more fun and pass quicker, we made everything a game. It was always "how many bags of cement can you carry?" We'd load each other up and then, straining under the bags, would try to make the others trip or drop their bags.

Making everything a game passed the time and made dull work fun. Adding that element of humor was an important lesson that we learned early from dad. Keeping your sense of humor would be one of the most important and needed lessons of my life. And I had a lot of occasions to use it.

My mother worked hard, too, but she didn't laugh as much. She was part Irish and part French-Canadian. Her French-Canadian father was born in a log cabin and her Irish relatives came to the United States because of the potato famine. Not so much laughing there!

But mom worked extremely hard. I learned from her and dad that hard work is a great thing. I remember once she was putting the clothes through a ringer to dry them and her hand got caught in the mechanism. Luckily the ringer had a catch for this very reason that stopped the mechanism. If it hadn't, it would have crushed and ruined her hand.

After she pulled her hand out, she stopped work, sat to the side, and cried for about 20 minutes. She cried hard, finished crying, and then went right back to work. Of course, I'd be in the hospital if something like that happened to me, but she was tough. I picked up some of her toughness and her perseverance. Believe me, that got me through later.

Mom stayed home and took care of the cleaning, cooking, and childcare. I remember how hard she worked, washing the clothes, the floor, cooking, and canning food for the coming winter. It seemed to never end for her. I guess I didn't help her because one of my favorite times was when she would sit me on the counter with my feet in the sink and wash me. She never minded the distraction from her work and always ended my wash-up with a kiss and a hug. It's no wonder I was dirty all the time.

Mom was always waiting when we came home from school. She took care of us when we were sick with colds and other childhood problems. Mom's caring nature didn't end with her children. She never got tired of the wounded wildlife we brought home that needed tender loving care and medical treatment. Mom would do her very best to help these adopted wounded. Of course, we would have tested even the most skilled veterinarian with our baby birds, turtles, frogs, mice and even crows that we kept in large birdcages. By being there for us and for our zoo, she taught me compassion and the importance of helping those who aren't able to help themselves.

With Dad working and studying, Mom had to do most of the work at home. As we got older she shared her household responsibilities with us. My job was emptying the water pan under the icebox. I was usually a little too late checking it and the pan constantly overflowed. I tried hard not to spill any water on the way to the sink, often without much success, and I would hear from Mom's Irish side about it. That helped me learn not to leave things to the last minute. Even today I drive my wife Marie crazy by packing the car for trips two days ahead of time.

In my mother's later years she spent a lot of time with doctors and in the hospital. Instead of giving up, she would get mad at the situation. It was easy to get her "Irish" up. I'm like my Mom: every diagnosis of cancer got my "Irish" up and put me in the mood for a good fight. And I had to do a lot of fighting.

I fought my diseases and other difficulties and my brothers and sisters worked hard in their own rights. Combining my dad's work with theirs, A. Boilard Sons is still going strong,

69 years later at the time of this writing. I worked there, along with my children, for years. My brother Bobby now owns the business and his two sons are doing a good job running it to this day.

Just as my dad was able to start a business based on the trust of others, the business is prospering to this day because of trust. The lumberyard is within five miles of both a Lowe's and a Home Depot and you'd think it would have a hard time competing with those two giants, but it doesn't. In fact, sometimes those two buy from the family business. We're able to be so successful, despite the odds, because we have strong relationships with contractors. At our competition, contractors are treated like numbers. When contractors buy from A. Boilard Sons, they're treated with professionalism and their needs, preferences, and histories are known. This is a big help to them because if they're building more than one house or building at a time, they appreciate the service.

So, whether it's been in life, health, or business, we've all been able to draw on mom's perseverance and toughness and dad's sense of humor to get us through. That sense of humor has been with me throughout my fights with cancer. Laughter, mine and others, has been a big factor in my survival and has been a friend when I faced other challenges. All the chemo and heart attacks and other hardships I've had might have damaged my health or dampened my spirits but they could never touch my humor.

Chapter 2
Surviving Drowning

S wimming was one of my favorite things to do growing up, even though I wasn't a strong swimmer. My friends and I would swim all over the place, in rivers and ponds and lakes. One place we swam a lot was the Chicopee River. We used to swim in a little area on that river protected from general view by trees. We called the nook BAB – Bare Ass Beach. You can probably guess from the name that the only bathing suits we wore there were the ones we were born in.

Sometimes when we'd swim there, girls would come and steal our clothes while we were in the water. Because I was the smallest, my friends always made me get out of the water and chase after the girls to get our clothes back. Oh, how they would scream and run away.

Even though it was dangerous, we'd find places to jump off rocks and bridges and things like that. And though those were the dangerous moments, my first brush with death came in a much less risky place, when I was around eleven years old.

I was a regular kid, spending a lot of time just having fun with my buddies. It was summer and summer meant

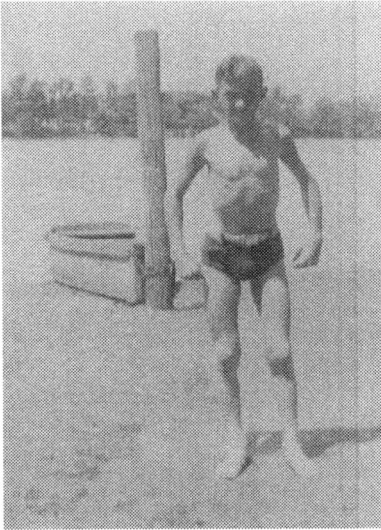

Because I was the smallest, my friends always made me get out of the water and chase after the girls to get our clothes back.

swimming. Though we liked the Chicopee River and BAB, our favorite place to swim was five miles away from my home at Havilland Pond in Ludlow. Five miles was too far to walk and of course we didn't have a car, so we rode our bikes. My friend Roland would let me sit on the back rack of his bike and put my feet on the peddles with his feet on top of mine. We both pedaled, doubling the horsepower, making it an easy trip to the pond.

One day, just like any other one that summer of 1935, we'd gone down to the lake to swim and picnic, carrying a lunch mom made us.

Like I said, I was not a strong swimmer. I just splashed and dogpaddled around near the shore, but never venturing with my friends out to the raft in the center of the pond, which seemed a long way off.

That day I thought I'd surprise my buddies and swim out to the raft where they already were. Without another thought off I went, keeping an eye on the raft at all times. I was paddling hard and getting tired, but the raft wasn't getting any closer. So I just paddled harder. Doing that only made me more tired.

I wasn't too close to the raft, but I was close enough that the waves made when the other kids jumped off into the water started crashing onto me. Between my tired muscles and the waves washing over me, I started to take in water and began to go under. For the first time in my life, but not for the last, I was starting to drown.

When I bobbed up from under the water for the third time, Roland saw that I was in trouble. He yelled for help from the lifeguard. Luckily, the lifeguard had seen what was happening and he was already in the water on his way to get me. He soon reached me and pulled me onto the raft.

I sat on that raft for a long time getting my breath back. Even though I'd almost drowned, I forced myself to get back into the water. I knew if I didn't do that I'd be too afraid to swim again. So after about an hour, I got into the water and dogpaddled back to shore. Somehow, the swim in that direction seemed much shorter.

When I go to Havilland Pond today, I have to smile at seeing how close the raft is to the shore.

I don't know how close I came to drowning but I realized that help from friends and professionals can keep your head above water. I learned to count on my friends to keep an eye on me, and that trained professionals, no matter the situation — whether it's drowning, money problems, or medical issues — should be called into action when you're in trouble.

Chapter 3
A Lesson From Basic Training

I liked school and I studied hard. I was never very good at grammar, and math turned almost impossible once we got to algebra, but I loved history and got good marks in it. I also had a real interest and aptitude in art.

After leaving middle school, I studied commercial art at the Springfield Trade School. After I had been there for three years World War II broke out and I was hearing constant stories about the war.

I was proud to be an American and loved my country. The government was using the stories from the war to make a lot of heroes and I ate those stories up. The ones I remember best were the Flying Tigers (more about them in a bit) and Capt. Colin Kelley. Kelley was a B17 pilot who was flying some bombers to Pearl Harbor the day the Japanese attacked. He tried to ram some of the Japanese planes in midair, to fight back, even though he had no ammunition because he was just transporting the planes. He was shot down and killed.

Hearing stories of that kind of heroism, and given how much I loved my country, convinced me that I wanted to go to war. My brothers felt the same way: All four boys served

Chapter 3: A Lesson From Basic Training

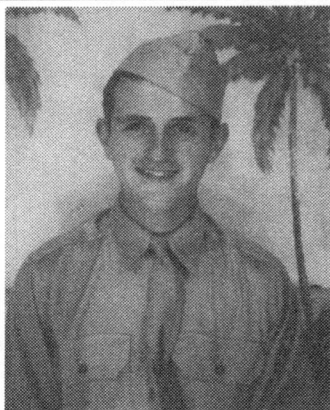

I wanted to join up so badly that I wrote to the one person who I thought would have the power to overrule every doctor in the country: President Franklin Roosevelt.

their country in time of war and we all made it home. Eddy volunteered for the Navy during World War II, even though he didn't have to go since he had a wife and two children. He spent many days at sea floating on a raft after his boat was sunk. Not long after D-Day, Billy went into Europe, where he was wounded and received a Purple Heart. My kid brother, Bobby, served in the Korean War. I served during World War II in the Army Air Force in India and Burma as ground crew and a flight engineer for a Douglas C-54 Cargo plane, carrying high-octane gas over the Himalayas for the B-29s bombing Japan. I had just turned 19.

I was proud to serve, but I almost didn't get the chance. I was very excited about the prospect of joining up so some friends and I went to volunteer. It turned out I was a little too excited. When it came to the physical, my heart was beating so hard and so fast that the doctor thought I had something wrong with me. Of course I didn't, I was just nervous and excited, but I failed the physical anyway.

Believe it or not, I actually failed three physicals.

I had dropped out of school to join the service and now that I had failed my physical, I wasn't sure what I was going to do. Eventually I decided to leave school permanently and my dad offered me a job at his business. Before I accepted, though, I gave the service one last shot.

I wanted to join up so badly that I wrote to the one person who I thought would have the power to overrule every doctor in the country: President Franklin Roosevelt. I never got a response from FDR, but someone must have seen the letter because it got passed to the Secretary of the Navy and he sent word to my local draft board that they ought to give me another shot at enlisting.

So I was called back in. But, boy, was I still nervous. The doctor performed my physical, but when he got to the heart check, my heart was still beating too hard. The doc told me to lie still and relax, and I did. He went away for a bit and then came back.

When he returned, he checked my heart again and finally I passed! This surprised me, but I was excited, too. The bigger surprise came when I was given my choice of what branch of the service I wanted to enter.

I had originally wanted to join the Navy, but since they hadn't seemed to want me after failing me in my physical so many times, I chose the Army.

I reported to Fort Devens, Massachusetts, after being inducted into the Army on – believe it or not! – April Fool's Day, 1943. That day the Sergeant asked for a volunteer to stoke the fires in the furnaces during the night. He said that the person who did this would have the next day off. Thinking I was pretty smart and would earn myself some extra rest, I stepped forward and volunteered. I spent the night taking care of the fires while sitting with the cook, eating and drinking coffee.

The next day I woke with a big smile on my face, thinking

that the others would have a full day on the drill field and I would get to stay in bed. I was pretty confused when no one got out of their bunks, though. I asked my bunkmate why no one was getting up and he replied, "Today's Sunday. Everyone has it off."

Monday morning I put my nose up against the sarge's nose, and thanked him for teaching me not to ever volunteer for anything in the Army.

I'd learned that if they wanted me they would call out my name. It's good to learn from your first experiences and stick to them. I never volunteered again.

Chapter 4
Surviving the Broken-Down Plane

When I joined the Army, I was sure I'd be fighting in the infantry, but I was put into the Army Air Force instead (the Air Force didn't become its own branch of the service until 1947. At the time it was part of the Army). Though I started training at Fort Devens, I finished in Miami Beach, which wasn't too hard to take.

I was assigned to become an airplane mechanic due to my IQ test, but I still wanted to fight and applied to become a gunner on a bomber. I was denied. They told me they had enough gunners already.

So I was sent to maintenance school in Biloxi, Mississippi, and then continued my warm-weather tour in San Diego where I worked at the Consolidated Aircraft plant where they made the B-24 bomber. Things in San Diego were pretty different: because Consolidated was providing food to the servicemen, we got five-course meals every night. Hard to argue with that, and better than any mess hall.

After San Diego I was shipped to Pueblo, Colorado, with a B-24 outfit. They put me in a service job, directing planes visiting the field to their parking spots. This wasn't a tough

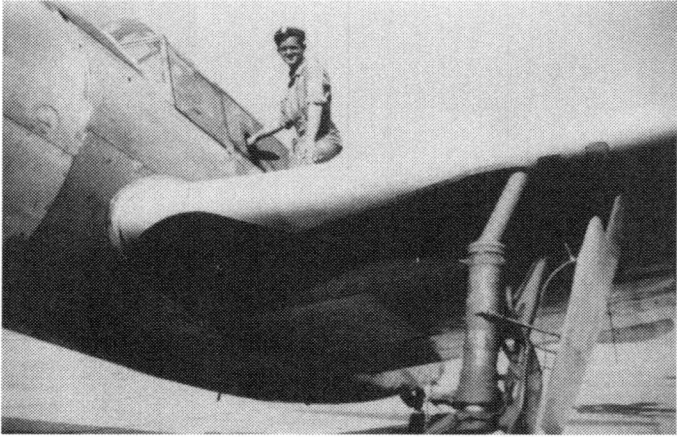

George Brown, our flight engineer and my friend, was teaching me how to be an engineer and we went a lot of places together.

job, but some of the pilots took me closer to death than I cared to be while still stateside!

When a plane landed it was my job to drive out in a jeep with this big sign on the back so the pilot could see I wanted him to follow me for parking. Some of the pilots stayed right on my backside because they thought it was funny. Well, I didn't think so – having four high-powered engines breathing down your neck is never fun and it was especially frightening at night! I'd always drive the planes to their parking spots quickly, and I'd catch hell from operations for going so fast. I made it my policy to reply to their complaints as soon as I changed my shorts and showered down.

My unit from Pueblo shipped to Italy without me. I had assumed I would go wherever they went, but it didn't turn out that way. Italy was terrible for them. They lost three quarters of the planes on their first raid.

Soon enough, I was deployed to India. I thought this was great because I was a Flying Tiger man at heart and had been since before I enlisted when the government was making heroes of them. The Flying Tigers were a group of about 100 pilots that the Army had secretly sent to Burma to help the Chinese protect roads and trade routes from the Japanese. People know them today for the shark tooth design they painted on the front of their planes. By 1942 they weren't a secret anymore and we all loved them.

But by the time I got out there in 1943, the Flying Tigers had been folded back into the Army Air Force. The new name of the unit was the 14th Air Force Squadron. I was disappointed that I wouldn't get to serve with The Flying Tigers, but the 14th kept the shark's teeth painted on their planes. Even though it wasn't quite like the old days, it felt good to have them flying with us, ready to provide cover, even if the air was empty of Japanese planes. Thanks to them, our only worries were the weather and The Hump, which is what we called the Himalayas.

George Brown, our flight engineer and my friend, was teaching me how to be an engineer and we went a lot of places together. We would often fly into China with 50-gallon drums of high-octane fuel. During one trip (and it just goes to show that being around airplanes was always dangerous for me!), after we'd unloaded and were ready to head home, George told me to take over the controls. I did as he said and took us up. As our wheels left the runway, he told me to lift the plane's flaps. I did, except I was supposed to milk them up five degrees at a time. I hadn't done it right and I got this big slap on the head from George. It was easy to see why: I looked out the front window to see that we were headed for a line of trees.

Luckily the pilot took over and pulled back on the stick. We cleared the trees and I made sure I milked the flaps from then on.

One day, George and I were assigned to fly into a Burmese airfield that the British had for their fighters. One of our planes, number 165, was down there and in need of repair. We were being sent to get it back into flying shape. We left India as passengers, riding in a general's C-47 that had been converted into a posh, deluxe plane. The only tools we carried were a hammer, pliers, safety wire, an adjustable wrench, and two screwdrivers - all in a toolbox no bigger then a briefcase, though it was fatter.

We landed in Burma and were taken to our plane. It was in bad shape: Three out of the four engines had something wrong with them. The magnetos – which powered the engine's sparkplugs to ensure that the plane would be able to fly even if there was a total electrical failure - were out of sync in the first engine. The prop control cable in engine two was broken, putting it at risk of becoming a runaway engine. Engine four had pushed its piston off the threaded bolts that held it down and the wing was covered in oil, top to bottom. Only engine three was in good shape, which was lucky since that's where the hydraulic pump was.

Even though we didn't have much to work with - not our normal set of tools, not a lot of technical support - George and I tackled the job. We went at engine four first, hammering the head down on the stripped bolts, using them like rivets to hold the thing in place. We washed and cleaned the engine.

Number two engine was next and we didn't have any cable to replace the broken prop control. All we had was some heavy Manila string, so we wrapped it tight and hoped for the best.

Engine one was the hardest to fix because we had no instruments to test the magnetos. We had to fix them by feel alone. So we'd fire up the engine, tweak it, and do it again to make sure that the engines fired together. If one fired ahead of the other, you'd get a rough ride on the engine.

By the time we were done, we weren't too sure that the whole thing would fire, let alone fly, but at least it looked good. That was something. We had the plane in the best condition we could manage.

Not long after, a jeep pulled up with two young pilots in it. One pilot – a lieutenant who, I think, was about six months younger than me – was going to have to fly the thing back over The Hump, so he came to me after we fired up the engines and asked me, "How's the plane?"

The best I could give him was, "Eh, OK."

I guess that didn't convince him, so he asked "if we take it up, will you come along?" I looked at George. He looked at me. We said sure. That made the pilot feel good enough to fly.

We got in the plane and I told the pilot that he might not want to pre-flight. If he did, he would have had to rev the engines to full power and I wasn't sure they'd make it.

He took my advice, skipped the pre-flight and we got off the ground. As we were going up, the pilot started to feather engines two and four, which is where you shut down the engines and turn the prop in them so that it doesn't windmill or create drag on the plane. We were flying on just two engines and the radio started cackling. The British control tower was squawking at us.

"Come back," they were saying. "You're in trouble!"

We had to get the plane back to India, so the pilot just shut off the radio. If he'd talked to them and then we'd crashed, he'd have gotten a hell of a hard time from our superiors – if we lived, that is!

We were flying fine, as far as we could tell, but we weren't real high off the ground. It seemed my optimism came a little too quickly, though, because soon enough the pilot told us to strip the cargo out of the plane. We got everything out – the cargo doors, the flare guns, everything we could find to make it lighter.

We were down so low that as we threw the cargo out, we scared up a herd of wild elephants. They were running like hell through the trees – going really fast. What a sight that was!

Even though we should probably have been worried about making it back to our airstrip, it never occurred to me or George. We were just having fun, having an adventure. We did have a moment's pause, though, when we realized that we couldn't abandon the plane if we needed to – we'd thrown out the parachutes! Not that it would have made a difference — we were too low to use parachutes anyway.

As we approached the landing strip, the pilot started engines two and four. Then he took us up to get some more altitude before landing. As he did, I looked down at the field and got my first good look at the sight that was assembled below. The field was covered in fire trucks and ambulances and there was a large white circle with a red cross inside it on the ground.

"We can't land, sir!" I shouted to the pilot.

"Why not," he asked and I pointed to the ground.

"Somebody's in trouble down there," I told him.

He looked at me and smiled. He knew what was going on, even though I didn't: we were the ones in trouble. All those people below us were there in case we crashed, which must have seemed pretty likely to them.

"Get your back against bulkhead six," the pilot shouted to George and me. "Pitch your back against it and hang on!"

We did what he said and he landed the plane. It was a beautiful landing, coming down without a hitch.

I learned later that the pilot hadn't been quite as confident as he'd let on (and to think that my vote of confidence in our repair job didn't convince him!): he'd radioed ahead to the field that we were only on two engines and that they should watch out for us.

It was funny, but I never had an inkling that we were in any trouble at all, let alone how much trouble we really were in. Neither did George. It just felt routine. We were in some pretty bad trouble, I guess, but we didn't notice. That's a gift of youth mixed with boundless optimism.

And that wasn't the only dicey experience I had in a plane while I was in Asia. There were some officers at the base who needed to get flight time in to keep their flight qualification and to stay at a certain pay level. To accommodate them, we had some Grumman planes with a lot of their combat gear, especially the weapons, taken out. Included in the removed items were some of the cockpit communications equipment, so the pilot wasn't able to talk to the person riding in the seat behind him.

One day I asked one of these officers if I could go up with him on his qualifying flight. He said sure. I climbed up the ladder after him and eased myself down between the metal bars, into the cockpit, and onto the seat, which, back then, doubled as a parachute.

He took us up and we were moving along nicely. Part of his qualification on the flight was to run a series of tests. One of these tests was to draw back on the throttle sharply and cause the plane's emergency horn to blow. Well, because there was no in-cockpit communication gear in the plane, I didn't know he was going to do this. So, when he pulled back on the throttle and the horn sounded, I thought something was seriously wrong with the plane.

I did what anyone would do when there's a problem with their plane: I tried to bail out. Hundreds of feet up in the air, in a plane going hundreds of miles an hour, I opened the canopy and prepared to parachute out! To make matters worse (in my mind, at least), I was stuck. I couldn't get out of my seat.

I knew the officer wouldn't bail out of the plane while I was still in it, so I was worried that if I didn't get out, he wouldn't either and we'd both be toast. But there I was, stuck.

He righted the plane and the horn stopped sounding and I realized that I didn't need to bail out. If I'd been able to, though, I would have parachuted out and that officer would have landed with one fewer passenger than he'd taken off with!

Despite spending so many years in the war and having a few adventures, I never saw any combat. I was lucky not to have seen any, to say nothing of not having been in D-Day or a similar battle, like my brother Billy was. I wasn't afraid of combat and I didn't avoid it, but it just never came my way.

Sometimes I'd talk to servicemen who'd just come back from battle and they would always wonder how they survived. The old saying they'd use was "the bullet didn't have my name on it." Whenever someone said this in front of me, I'd always reply, "Yes, but what about the ones marked 'To Whom It May Concern?'" I had a fatalistic view of the whole thing, you see. I thought I wasn't going to make it home.

I used to go to confession to Father O'Brien. We'd be out in a field and he'd have a pair of folding chairs to use as a makeshift confessional. I'd go to him and say things like "I got real pruned last night, Father. I drank too much."

"Chick," he'd say to me, "you're going home, you're going to have a family. You've got to think of them."

I'd look at him and say, "Who? Me, Father? I'm not going to make it. I'm not going to make it."

I truly felt I wouldn't get back home because I believed that I'd never done anything to deserve God getting me through the war. But I got through. And I guess maybe what we did at the orphanage might have earned me some brownie points.

Chapter 5
The Importance of Charity: The Orphanage

When I was stationed in India, I spent some time at an airbase at the foot of the Himalayas called Tesgan. At the base I used to pal around with a pair of guys. I didn't know their names, really, and I don't know if they knew mine. But the three of us were good friends: The Polack, the Russian, and me, Frenchie. That's what we called each other. We'd all go out together when we weren't on duty. We especially liked to spend our free time going into the town and having Japanese rice wine, sake, which we liked to mix with Orange Crush soda.

At Christmastime, the Red Cross came in and had a party for the GIs and the three of us went. They had a bunch of children with them from a local orphanage.

During the party, the nun who ran the orphanage told all the GIs that if we were ever going to buy any jewelry, we should come down to the orphanage to do it, because they had a store and the money would help the children. So I told the Polack and the Russian that we might as well do it, since they could use the money. They agreed.

We went down to the orphanage one day to buy some

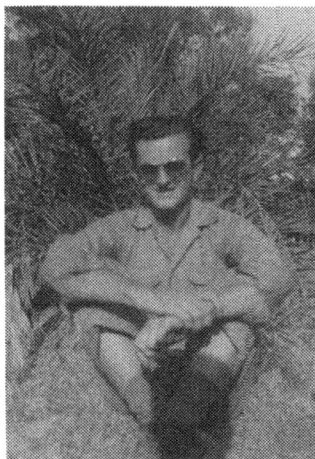

When I was stationed in India, I spent some time at an airbase at the foot of the Himalayas called Tesgan.

jewelry and to my surprise they didn't actually have a store. They just had a dealer who would come to the orphanage to sell to other people after the nun went and got him. I had thought that maybe the kids were making the jewelry themselves or something like that, so this wasn't the arrangement I was expecting. I didn't like it, so we didn't buy anything.

Before we left, the nun cornered us. She was quite the politician and had a plan for us, I think. She asked us if we'd like to see the orphans. We said sure.

She took us to a classroom where the kids — all little girls — were learning. They looked up at us when we entered. They were staring at us, so young and with these innocent little eyes, and the scene just broke my heart. They were writing on these little slate boards with wooden frames, just like Abraham Lincoln did almost 100 years before. I asked the sister why they were using them.

"Because we don't have any paper," she said.

I didn't think this was right and I had an idea about how we could fix it. I went back to the base and immediately wrote my father. Then as now, salesmen like to leave behind little trinkets with their company's name on them and so my dad got a lot of pads of paper and pencils and the like from salesmen. And just like now, he didn't need them all. So I wrote and asked him to send all the pads and pencils that he could get his hands on. It must have been a weird letter — I didn't even tell him why I wanted them. He never wrote back, though, and never asked me what I wanted them for, so I forgot about it among all the other activity.

But then, two or three months later, a big package arrived for me at the base. It took so long to get there because it had to come by boat and it had gotten pretty banged up on the trip. All the guys thought someone had sent me a cake (well, maybe they were wishing for it more than really thinking it), but after a trip like that a cake would have been ruined.

I opened the box and found a big stack of pads of paper and a bunch of pencils from my dad. I grabbed my friends and told them that we ought to go bring them to the sister and the children right away.

We knocked on the door and the sister opened it to find me holding a big box.

"Here," I said. "This is for the kids."

Boy was she was thrilled. She grabbed two pads of paper and three pencils and ran around saying, "The kids are going to write!" She had tears in her eyes.

After a little while of this, she asked us to stay and eat with the children. We told her that we didn't want to eat their food, but she insisted that we stay. We again tried to beg off eating the children's food, but she kept up, so eventually we gave in. Of course, it turned out that she had another reason for wanting us to stay. Like I said, she was a real politician — and a good one at that.

Because they were all they had, the kids ate at the same desks where they took their studies and so when we went to eat with them, we had to sit in the desks, too. So there we were, three big gawky guys, overflowing out of these little children's desks. The nun came around serving the food and laid a bowl of clear, soapy-looking water and a piece of bread in front of us.

I could hardly believe it. I looked at her and asked, "Is this all the kids have to eat?"

She said that it was.

I swallowed that answer and soaked my bread in the water. It didn't taste very good. I couldn't believe that was all these poor kids had to eat. Times were tough for us growing up during the Depression, but they were never that tough.

The scene stuck in my mind, but I didn't see what I could do about it.

A few days later, I was in the mess hall at the base and watched as some of the guys came into the kitchen and helped themselves to some food. Suddenly I had an idea. I turned to the cook, who, like every cook everywhere, we called Cookie, and asked him what he did with the food we didn't eat in the mess hall.

"Why, we throw it away," he said.

"Throw it away?" I asked, surprised. "Why don't we give it to the kids at the orphanage?"

"That's a damn good idea," said Cookie, "but I can't do it. You've got to see the base commander."

And so we did. I rounded up the Polack and the Russian and we got all dressed up — pressed our pants, shined our shoes — and went to see the base commander.

Well, he took one look at us and got suspicious.

"What do you guys want?" he asked, eyeing us.

I stepped forward and told him that the kids at the local orphanage had nothing to eat and that we wanted to give them the uneaten food from the mess hall.

He thought it was a great idea and gave us the go ahead right away. He just told us to make sure that the sister gave our metal pots back, because we needed those to feed the base.

So pretty soon we got our first load together and went back to the orphanage with all kinds of pots of food. We had mashed potatoes, carrots, peas, everything. God, the sister was excited!

We started to bring the food to her on a regular basis, which she appreciated. And the best part was still to come.

We didn't really say anything about what we were doing to anyone else at the base because we weren't looking for anyone's thanks. We just wanted to do something good for someone else. But somehow the guys found out.

Most nights, we had a fruit cocktail for dessert. After a while, though, we started to notice that no one was eating the fruit cocktail anymore. I came to find out that somehow the other guys at the base had heard about what we were doing for the orphanage and had decided not to eat the fruit cocktail so it could be given to the kids. Seeing what those guys did, without even being asked, made me feel pretty good.

Doing the right thing, doing a nice thing, for someone else when you can makes you feel so good. I never did something charitable because I wanted something in return, but I always found good came my way — even if it was just a good feeling — when I did. If there is a God, and I believe there is, I think it can only help us with Him. And maybe doing that kind of good thing is part of why I made it through so many scrapes with death and am here to tell you these stories today.

Chapter 6
Hunting The Phantom Tiger

George and I were given some R & R time on the beaches of Burma. We were flown in on a C-47 that landed on the beach when the tide was out. We spent our days wearing just jockstraps, shell belts, carbines, helmets, and combat boots. What a sight we were, two skinny white guys playing in the sun, getting as tan as the natives.

One day we decided to go walking through the jungle, to explore. As George and I were taking in the sights, we saw dozens of flying squirrels coasting through the air above us.

"Geez, I bet it would be hard to shoot one of those guys," George said.

I figured he was right and let it go.

We kept walking and after a bit came upon the most beautiful swimming hole. It looked like it should have been in a Tarzan movie. We splashed around there for a while, not really going swimming but enjoying the area, until we saw a few big animal tracks in the mud. They were just the right size and shape to belong to a tiger.

We decided to leave, but we both agreed that we'd be back. We were going to hunt that tiger.

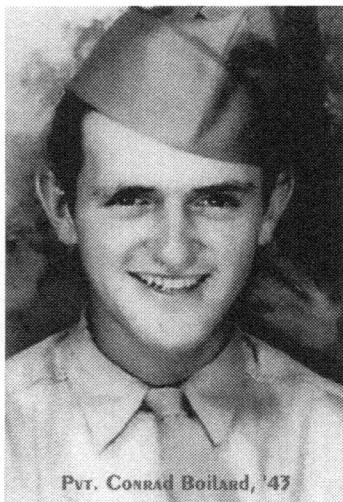

PVT. CONRAD BOILARD, '43

We decided to leave, but we both agreed that we'd be back. We were going to hunt that tiger.

So we headed back to the camp and went to see the superior officers. We told them our plan: that we wanted to bag a tiger.

"Sure," they said, if you can believe it. "Go ahead."

We equipped ourselves with rifles – fittingly, I had a bolt-action Springfield rifle — and a flashlight and headed out into the night.

We waited by the swimming hole for a while, but no tiger. Eventually it got so dark — and believe me when I say it got dark in the jungle, dark like you've never seen; we really needed that flashlight! — that I told George we ought to give up for the night and head back to camp.

He agreed and we got going. To get out, we had to squeeze through a really narrow area between two rocks. It was so thin that we needed to turn sideways and hold our rifles in front of us just to fit through. George was behind me, but he was carrying the flashlight to show the way.

We were about halfway through when suddenly George

fired his rifle! I got through that pass faster than his bullet and George was right behind me.

"Why the heck did you fire?" I shouted.

"I saw the flashlight reflect in a pair of eyes," he said. "They were looking right down on us from the rocks."

He thought it was the tiger and so he shot. As far as I know, he missed.

Believe it or not, it was only then that I got nervous. It hadn't occurred to me before then that what we were doing was all that dangerous. Just like in the plane: only after it was over did I understand how truly dangerous things were. That night, I could have ended up as supper for a tiger.

Chapter 7
Almost Roadkill

Growing up in Indian Orchard, we had a motorcycle mechanic living just up a hill behind us. He didn't have enough room in his garage to do all the work he needed, so he'd often take the engines out of the bikes to work on in his shop. He'd leave the gutted motorcycles outside next to his garage.

The motorcycles were mostly useless without their engines, but we found ways to put them to use. At night we'd sneak up the hill to his shop and have some fun with those bikes. We'd take turns getting on them and having others push us down the hill, coasting down and just have a great time. And no one ever got hurt.

So, by the time I got to Burma I was used to clowning around with cars and the like. Unlike when I was young, though, in Burma it came back to bite me.

One day we were headed to the range for target practice. There were a bunch of us, all piled onto a 6 X 6 Army truck. I'd been over there for a while at this point and I thought I was a real big shot. To show just how big I was, I was riding on the front winch of the truck in my standard jungle uniform:

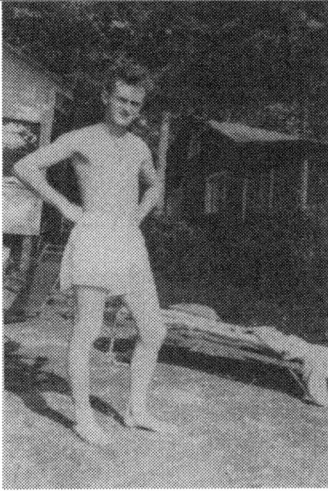

To show just how big I was, I was riding on the front winch of the truck in my standard jungle uniform: jock strap, combat boots, gun belt, helmet, and my carbine in my left hand.

jock strap, combat boots, gun belt, helmet, and my carbine in my left hand. I was holding onto the truck with my right hand.

As we drove, we came across a river flowing out of the jungle. I never found out the river's name, but after what it did to me, I wish I had.

The water was wide and deep. Someone, it seems, thought that it would be funny to drive hard into the water to try to soak me. Our driver hit the gas and in we went. And boy did I get wet! In fact, the plan worked too well: I went flying off the winch and into the water. The deep, fast water was rushing all around me and the truck was driving over me and I thought, not for the last time in my life, "well, this is it."

There's the cliché that your life flashes in front of your eyes when you're about to die. It did anything but for me; time seemed to slow down. The first thing I did was what many Catholics would have done: I said an Act of Contrition. I then thought of my Mom and Dad, my brothers and sister. I quickly made a list of who owed me money and to whom I owed money. All this in the few seconds in the water while the truck was driving over me.

As the truck got over me, my mind sped up quickly and my new concern was that the rear end of the truck was going to catch my helmet and drag me along the river bottom. If that happened, I knew I wouldn't be able to hold my breath long enough and that I'd drown.

But instead of catching my helmet, the truck ran over me, its inside set of dual tires on me, with the outside set on some nearby rocks. The driver stopped the truck. I yelled inside my head, "Get this damn truck off of me!" Maybe somehow someone heard me because at that moment the truck moved and I could see the sun shining through the water.

I tried to stand but my legs were too weak to hold me. I started to fall and the sergeant caught me before I could slip back into the river.

They drove me back to camp and went looking for the doctor. When they found one and he examined me, he turned me over on my belly and said that I had tire marks on my left fanny cheek and left leg. What a sight I must have been – just like a cartoon.

The doctor told me that I might have a problem sleeping that night because of the injuries, so he gave me six sleeping pills. I thought I wouldn't need them because I was a good sleeper, but he was right. After hours of tossing and turning, I took all six pills and went out hard and fast.

The next morning, the boys were going to breakfast and they came to check in on me. When they woke me, I found I couldn't move a muscle and I could barely talk. They lifted me out of bed, dragged me to the mess hall and held me up so I could have breakfast. I was told that I would have to see a doctor back at our main base because the doctor at the camp didn't have the right equipment to help me. So, despite not being able to walk more than a few limping steps, I was on my own until I got back.

Once we got back to base, I limped for about a month and was unable to perform my regular duties. Doctor's orders, of course. I was left all alone when the rest of the guys went back to work.

One day some of my buddies rushed into the barracks where I was staying to tell me our plane, number 165, was on fire. I was concerned about the crew and started to limp as quickly as I could — which was pretty slow — to the base, seven miles away. Along the way, an airman in a jeep picked me up. He dropped me off at the apron of the hangar where the plane was burning. At the sight of the burning plane I forgot my injuries and started to jog, and then run, to the scene.

Luckily, my crew was all right. Rather than being hurt, they were surprised. They all just stared at me. Benny, our crew chief, called me a faker. After seeing me run like that he couldn't believe that I had truly been hurt. I think the running caused me to lose my limp, though, which I was glad of.

More than once I've asked myself what I learned from this trouble and the answer is not clear. Sometimes these things are clear right away, sometimes they never are. Still, my belief in a higher power, a guardian angel, or whatever you may believe in, was strengthened by this experience. Someone or something made sure I survived, was pulled out of the water, wasn't crippled. This made me even more sure that God does exist. Stay quiet and you'll hear Him.

Chapter 8
Love Lessons

When I was overseas I wrote a lot of letters to the girls back home. These girls were all people I'd grown up with. There had been a group of us in Indian Orchard, maybe 6 or 8 girls and 6 or 8 boys, who had always hung around together, though nothing really ever happened between any of us. They were simpler times, after all.

So I wrote letters to a lot of girls and I wrote about the same subject to each of them. I didn't do it because I was trying to play games with them or be smart; I did it because there were only so many things I was allowed to write about. Writing about the war or fixing airplanes was strictly off limits. If I'd tried to write about that stuff, the military censors would have cut it.

Well, one day the girls got together and started comparing the letters I'd sent them. They quickly realized I'd sent them all the same letter.

After this discovery, most of them stopped writing back — except for one, named Marie Ladue. We had been in the same group of friends and belonged to the same church. My

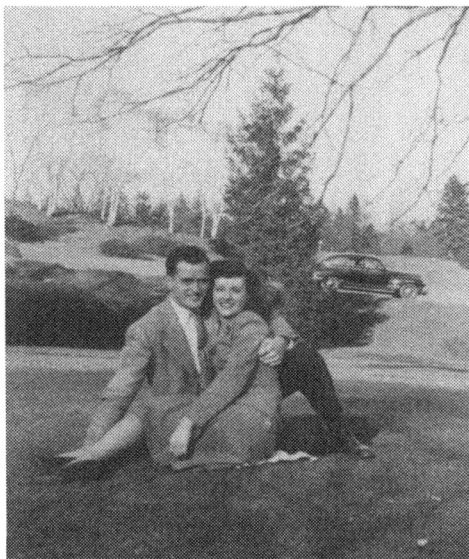

I was about to give up, figuring she just didn't want to see me, but as I was going to hang up, she said, "give me an hour, OK?" I gave her 55 minutes and drove to her home on Worcester Street.

confidence in getting anywhere with Marie was low because I was bowlegged, but she kept writing, even though we'd never had anything serious between us and weren't writing anything mushy.

She was a beautiful girl and I'd always tried to make time with her, even if nothing else was going to happen.

In the letters I wrote her, I would draw little pictures and icons to try to spice things up and make up for the fact that I wasn't allowed to write about the exciting parts of being at war. So we kept our letters on the lighter side. Marie sent me a photo of herself and we kept in touch.

I was really happy to be writing to someone, but I was also happy that it wasn't so serious, either. I saw a lot of guys get their hearts broken while they were overseas. They'd rushed to get married before shipping out — some of them didn't even have a chance to consummate the marriage — and then, after

49

they'd been overseas a while, they'd get a "Dear John" letter. I was glad that wasn't going to happen to me.

Marie and I wrote the entire time I was gone. The letters weren't any great shakes, we never said "I love you" in them, but she kept those letters tied up in ribbons and our daughters read them in their youths. What a treasure!

When I got discharged in February 1946, we were shipped back to California and mustered there. After that they put us Eastern boys on a train and sent us back to Massachusetts.

When the train stopped at the Springfield Railroad station I called home and said that I'd be going by the house, which was near the tracks, and I would try to wave. My family was surprised and happy that I was in the area. Well, as I came near the old Indian Orchard station, the other soldiers opened the window and had me lean out while they held my legs.

As we went by the house and lumberyard, it was like a Norman Rockwell painting. It was February and cold, and there was snow on the ground. I had tears in my eyes and I waved like hell to everybody I could see. Mom was on the front porch and waving for all she could. Dad was on his way to get the mail, and stopped the car, leaving the motor running, and got out to wave. Alex, our yard foreman, and the office help were out waving, too. The workers were on the station platform waving, my brother Billy was waving. It was one of the most memorable scenes in my life. I was sure happy to be home.

Once I was back, though, the first news I heard broke my heart. I was told that Marie was engaged. I was home for three days with my mind not in tune after I heard that. One Saturday I was in the office, and I picked up the phone and called Marie. She answered and I congratulated her on her engagement. Her reply? "I'm not engaged to anyone."

Well both feet hit the floor and I asked her if I could come down and see her. Her first reaction was "No." She said she wasn't ready to see me. Her hair wasn't done and she wasn't dressed well enough for me. I told her I didn't care how she looked, that I wanted to see her. She was persistent and I was about to give up, figuring she just didn't want to see me, but as I was going to hang up, she said, "give me an hour, OK?" I gave her 55 minutes and drove to her home on Worcester Street, parked on the wrong side of the road, ran up the front steps, and rang the doorbell.

She opened the door.

There stood the most beautiful girl in the world.

When I saw Marie, you could have hit me with a Louisville Slugger. My mouth dropped open, I couldn't move. Luckily, she asked me in. In one of my letters I had written that I was going to hug and kiss her when I saw her, so she had told her parents to stay out of the living room. But I didn't touch her. I didn't want to bust the dream I was having at the moment.

We started dating soon after that. Marie and I did the normal stuff while we were dating: We'd go to a movie, see big bands play when they came to town. We'd do things with our old gang of friends, too, but it was never quite the same as it had been before we went to war.

Despite spending all this time together, I wasn't very sure of myself on account of my bowlegs. I'd been turned down by girls so many times I felt like a bed sheet and
I was pretty self-conscious.

So when I started to think about asking Marie to marry me, I wasn't confident at all that I'd get a positive answer. As a result, I didn't plan any big event or to-do when I asked her.

51

In fact, I hadn't even bought a ring. After all, I didn't want to spend the money on a ring if she was just going to say no. What good was a ring going to do me without a girl to wear it?

One day I said to her, "If I buy you a ring, will you wear it?"

She thought about it for a minute and said, "Sure, I'll wear it."

We'll celebrate our 60th wedding anniversary on July 27, 2006.

After she said yes, I went to the city to buy her a ring. I didn't really believe in jewelry like that, but that's what was expected, so I did it.

Even so, I wasn't planning to buy anything expensive. I went to see a jeweler and got a good deal on a slightly damaged ring that a showcase had fallen on. I felt like I'd done my job.

I knew I was wrong when I got home. When my mom saw the ring, boy was she mad! She didn't think it was right that I give that ring to Marie. So the next day she dragged me by the ear back to the jeweler and read that jeweler the riot act. When we left, I had a new ring for Marie – one that cost me twice as much!

Even though we'd agreed to be married, we hadn't set a date. We got to it one night when we were out dancing with our friends Helen and Jerry, who were getting married, too. Helen and I were talking about my marriage to Marie and her marriage to Jerry Morneau. I told her that we were planning to get married in a year, since I'd only been home for about six months.

We got to talking and decided it would be better to get married on the same day in July, which was only a few months later. I asked Marie and she agreed.

When Marie went home and told her mother, she asked, "what's the matter with him? Can't he wait?" meaning couldn't I wait for sex. Different times, remember.

"No, he can't!" answered Marie and so we got married that July. Except for one of my brothers, every member of my family, including my parents, has been married in July.

Marie truly is the best thing to ever happen to me. She gave me a wonderful family of two boys and two girls. I became a husband and father, and I was truly happy.

Marie was the big factor in fulfilling my many dreams: photography, travel, and most importantly, having a family.

Chapter 9
Family

Having a family was a big goal Marie and I shared and we wanted to get started on it as soon as we were married. But before we even got married, we started having a house built for the family we were planning. We built it with three upstairs bedrooms, which Marie always said was enough room for eight kids – four in each room, and one room for us. We didn't quite end up with that many, but we did OK.

Before I went to war, my dad had promised me that when I got back he'd get me going with a house. After we were married, he gave us some money to get us started and at the end of every year he paid $1,000 against the principal on our mortgage. He was a big help to us.

We were paying $76 a month on the mortgage, which was for $6,000. Building the house cost $14,000. Paying $14,000 for a house back then is like paying $300,000 for a house these days. We knew people who were paying $150 a month on their mortgage and we couldn't imagine how they could afford it.

We lived in that house for 38 years – all the years we were raising our family and some afterwards, too.

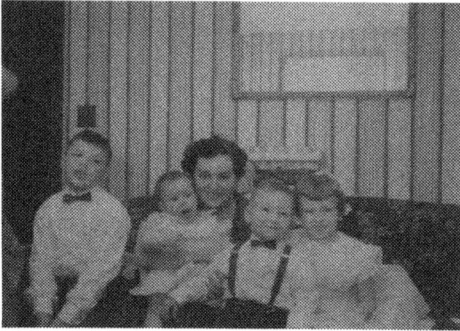

There was four years between the girls and four years between the boys. Christopher is our oldest son, born in 1950. Michelle is our oldest daughter, born in 1952. Then we had Mark in 1954 and finally Lynne in 1957.

After we were first married, we tried and tried to have kids (and the trying wasn't so bad!), but after about four years of marriage we didn't have any children to show for it, due to medical issues that made conception difficult. Some doctors even told us that we'd likely never have children. But we were determined to have a family, so we decided to adopt a child instead.

We were active in the church and asked the priests to work on our problem and see if they could find us a child to adopt. It took a while for them to find one. We had some near misses: we were two weeks late getting to a pair of twins, a boy and a girl. They had to break them up and give them to two families to get them adopted. We would have taken them both, which I think would have been better for them, but we were too late.

Finally, one day in 1950, we got a call and they told us they had a little boy we could adopt. We went down to the orphanage to see him and fell in love on the spot. He was so small, so young – he was just out of the hospital and still had his umbilical cord.

We brought him home and named him Christopher. Chris really changed our luck with children. After we adopted him, lo and behold, Marie became pregnant and we ended up with three of our own – two girls and another boy. There was four years between the age of the girls and four years between the boys. Christopher was born in 1950. Michelle is our oldest daughter, born in 1952. Then we had Mark in 1954 and finally Lynne in 1957.

Though getting married to Marie was the proudest moment of my life, being a father was a close second. What a wonderful thing it was. All of my love and concern went into the children and soon we did everything together as a family.

We went on vacations together, the kids worked in the lumberyard, and we all went to church. The first time we took Mark to church, he was very young. When the priest came out to light some of the candles near the altar, Mark saw them and started to sing "Happy Birthday to you!" And boy did he sing it loud. Everyone got a pretty good laugh out of that. For a while, Marie and I had to go to church in shifts because the kids were too young, but eventually we were able to go as a family.

There were two things I always wanted for the kids: to make sure they were good swimmers – not like their old man! – and for them to have good teeth. Well, they got both and I felt pretty good about that.

When we'd go on vacations, we'd often go swimming or on picnics. We'd take vacations with our friends, the Morneaus. We'd drive out to the Mohawk Trail for picnics or head to Enfield, Connecticut, and play cards on the picnic benches while the kids swam in the river.

This is what my parents did for us when we were kids, too. Of course it was the Depression back then and that was the only entertainment we had since there wasn't too much money, but still, we had a great time. We'd all pile into the pickup truck, Lillian in front with my parents and all the boys in the back, and head out. In the back, we'd spend the trip clowning around, waving to cars, and just having a great time.

Of course, we made sure that the kids learned the value of a hard day's work, too. That's how I grew up and I thought it was important that the kids got to work early and learned how to operate in that world.

We had my dad's lumberyard then, so as soon as the kids were old enough to get their working papers, we put them to work. Michelle and Lynne worked in the office, after school and on Saturdays. Mark and Chris worked out in the yard, painting fences and doing that sort of thing.

We paid the kids for their work and they got to keep their money. When Marie was growing up, she worked at a job and made $26 a week. When she took her pay home, $24 of it went to her mother. But we made sure the kids had their own money, so they could do things like go to the movies and could learn how to handle money. Of course, they were so busy that they hardly had time to spend it!

The kids never gave us any trouble, but we did have a medical issue with Mark early on: he had infant eczema, a terrible skin disease. It made his skin brittle and itchy, so he was constantly scratching it. It got so bad that you'd pick him up and when you put him down you'd have blood on your arms and clothes. We used to have to tie him down when he was sleeping so that he wouldn't scratch his skin and we would put splints on his arms when he was awake so he couldn't scratch. We had to lie awake nights watching him to prevent the scratching. We'd try to give him sleeping pills, but enough pills to put eight adults to sleep only knocked him out for 30 or 45 minutes!

We took him to the hospital in Springfield and he stayed there for a month. The doctor asked us to stop coming to visit because our arrival got Mark so excited that he'd move and scratch and cause himself more problems. No parent would like leaving their child alone in the hospital, but the doctor thought it was best, so we stayed away. By the end of that month, he was calling the doctor daddy!

We then took him to see a doctor in Boston who specialized in skin problems. That doctor took one look at him and said "no doctor north, south, east, or west is going to be able to cure this." It was the worst case he'd ever seen, he said, and asked our permission to take pictures of Mark so he could use them in teaching. He did tell us, though, that Mark was lucky to have gotten the eczema as a baby because he would likely outgrow it by the time he was five. If he had gotten it after five he probably would never have outgrown it.

The doctor gave us some pointers and a treatment to ease things and sent us home on a Friday. We gave Mark the treatment over the weekend and by Monday it was like he had a whole new skin: Everything was better and we couldn't believe it!

We took him to the doctor and after he examined him, he turned to us and said "this is not the child I examined last time." We assured him it was.

"I didn't do that," he said, meaning curing the problem. He was happy that it had been fixed, though.

Before we left one of the nurses pulled us aside and told us she thought God had helped Mark. She might have been right.

Even though we were very happy with our four children, some of whom were still younger than 10, we did eventually take in another child. Marie's aunt had adopted a girl a number

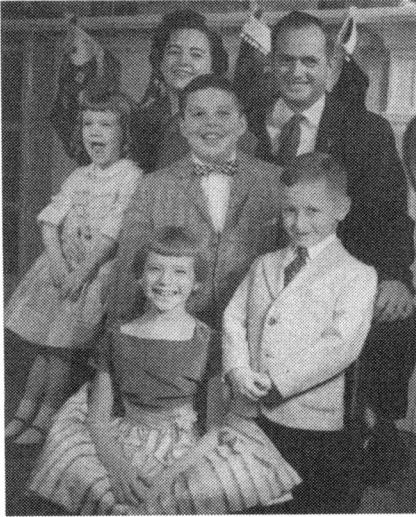

Though getting married to Marie was the proudest moment of my life, being a father was a close second. What a wonderful thing it was. All of my love and concern went into the children and soon we did everything together as a family.

of years before and by the early 1960s the girl was living with Marie's parents. Her parents were getting on in years – her father had rheumatoid arthritis and was on crutches and in bed a lot – and having a 13-year-old, as she was at the time, around was difficult for him.

So we took her into our home and she lived with us all through high school. After that, she went to live with her mother.

When she got married, she asked me to walk her down the aisle and give her away. I was the only real father figure she'd ever had. Of course I was glad to do it.

Because I took wedding pictures as a hobby, I was also her photographer. So I had to take pictures of the church, walk her down the aisle, run to the back and get my camera and take pictures of the ceremony! It was a busy day for me, but it was a wonderful day, too, and we were glad to have been a part of it.

After Mark's early health troubles were conquered, our kids grew up healthy and strong. I played some city league baseball at the time, even though I wasn't that good. The guys on the team knew I liked it, so they overlooked a lot of things and let me play a couple of innings at the beginning of the game. Of course, when the late innings rolled around and things got tight, I never saw the field, but that was OK with me.

Even though I wasn't so good, I tried to teach Mark and Chris how to play the game. And boy they got good. They could do all sorts of things on the field – the coaches loved having them on the team. Chris also played high school football. They both played pool, too.

One day they were going to a banquet to get trophies for winning some pool matches. They drove together and after the banquet were going to bring some friends by the house. Mark was 22 then, Chris 26. It was 1977.

On Marks' way home after dropping Chris off at his home, Mark's car struck a tree. He wasn't wearing a seatbelt. He was badly injured and was taken to the hospital. He went frequently in and out of consciousness and had many broken bones. Because he was so badly hurt, they could not operate on him immediately.

When he was in the hospital, no one knew whether he'd recover or not. Michelle came back from Worcester to be with him and Lynne, who was still living at home, went to visit him all the time.

At first he showed a lot of positive signs, moving when we talked to him, making noises. I remember Michelle coming home from visiting him once and telling Marie that she was sure Mark could hear her because he moved when she talked.

When he was in the hospital, I prayed to God. I told God

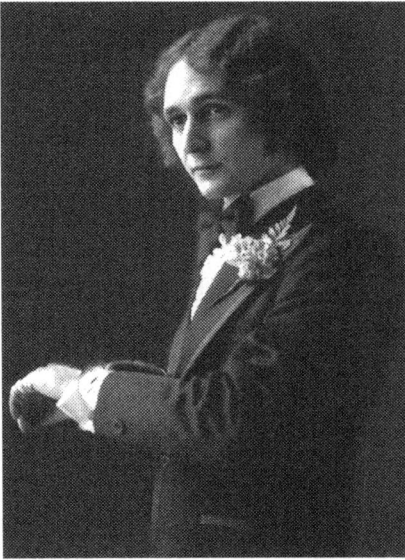

On Marks' way home after dropping Chris off at his home, Mark's car struck a tree. He wasn't wearing a seatbelt.

that I didn't care if he couldn't move, if he wasn't going to be the same. As long as I could communicate with him, I told God, that was enough. If we weren't going to be able to communicate, I prayed for God to take him.

At one point, a plastic surgeon brought me and Marie into his office and sat us down. He told us to pray that Mark die. He told us that every bone in his face was broken and that the longer he was in and out of consciousness the more the bones in his face would heal in their broken position. If that happened and he recovered, the surgeon told us they'd have to rebreak all of his facial bones to repair them. He told us that neither we nor Mark would want to go through that.

We never had to face that decision. There was some suspicion after a few days that he was brain dead. The doctors couldn't declare this, though, until he'd had three encephalograms to test his brain functions. He'd had two already.

On his ninth day in the hospital, the nurses were taking him for his third encephalogram and on his way to the test, he had a heart attack and died.

Lynne had been at the hospital that day visiting him. A doctor told her the news. She came home very upset, of course. Both of the girls took it very hard. Mark and Lynne were very, very close since Lynne still lived at home and Mark lived near us.

His loss was a terrible thing and we mourned for him. We knew we weren't the only parents ever to lose a child, but that didn't help any. Marie was able to go on because she had a job to go to. That was good for her. If she'd just sat home and mourned, it would have been harder.

I had seen a lot of death during the Depression and the war and so I knew you just had to go on, had to get through it. So I did. And we had three other children to worry about, too. If Mark had been our only child it would have been even harder, but we still had three to care for.

We didn't lose our faith or become bitter, though. Losing our son didn't stop us from going to church or from believing in God. That's the worst reason I can think of for not believing. Church and religion were only a help to us.

Our friends were great aids as well. The Morneaus came and stayed at our house for a while. Other friends would stop by or call to see how we were doing. It was another good time to have good friends.

Chapter 10
Surviving Non-Hodgkins Lymphoma

Working as a purchasing agent for the lumber company, I got to know the salespeople who called on me. One day in January 1975, a vendor named Bernie Barrett came to see me and as we sat and talked he mentioned that my neck was swollen on the right side. I told him that it wasn't and I pulled my head to the left and put my hand on my neck to check it out. I felt nothing unusual. Bernie insisted: "Chickie, your neck is swollen." I again put my hand to my neck but this time I kept my head straight. My heart dropped. I felt a large, firm lump.

I picked up the phone, called my doctor, Dr. Mazur, and told him what I had found. I was in his office the next day. I went into the hospital the day after that and was operated on that same day. My stay in the hospital lasted only a few days after that.

I got bored pretty quickly in the hospital. The second day I was there I pulled one of the nurses aside and asked her to get me a Manhattan, which was my favorite drink. She said she didn't have them.

I asked Marie for one, though, and one day she brought

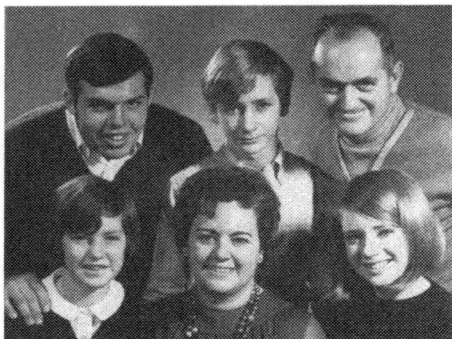

Cancer, the thinking went, meant you might have five years to live, tops. I went home and started to get my house in order. First thing I did was go to Confession. I needed to make peace with God.

me a little bottle of pre-mixed Manhattans. The same day some friends of ours came to the hospital.

Even to this day they say, "We came to see Chickie dying and there he was, making Manhattans!"

I left the hospital with a lot of questions. What I knew was that they took out a tumor that they thought had been growing slowly for years.

A week later, Marie and I went to see the doctor to get some answers. The biggest question was whether the tumor was cancerous or not. The doctor said it was cancer, Non-Hodgkin's Lymphoma. Lymphoma is a disease that affects the lymph nodes and Non-Hodgkin's Lymphoma is the most common kind, he told us.

The next question was whether the cancer had spread. The doctor told us it seemed to be confined to the tumor.

These days that would be good news, but back then nearly any cancer was seen as a death sentence. Cancer, the thinking went, meant you might have five years to live, tops. I went home and started to get my house in order. First thing I did was go to Confession. I needed to make peace with God. The second thing I did was have a will made. I needed to make sure I took care of my family.

Learning I had Lymphoma put me in deep thought. Doctor Mazur said it would be a good idea to have some radiation treatments on my neck as a safety valve to take care of any remaining cancer in the area. Arrangements were made for me at Wesson Hospital in Springfield. Not knowing what I would be facing, I was concerned about what was about to happen to me.

I drove to the hospital, parked the car in the lot, walked into the hospital, and went to the information desk to find out where I was to go. They sent me to the basement, of course. The scary things are always down in the basement. It was so dark down there that I could have used a flashlight. My heart was pumping like mad – just like when I was trying to pass my Army physical - as I walked down the stairs and into a large room. Inside were a doctor who ran the radiation machine and a nurse. She was cute, and I tried to kid with her, as I always do when facing problems, especially life or death problems.

They took me into a very dark room. They told me to sit in a chair that looked like the kind a dentist or barber uses. It was then that I noticed this monster of a machine pointing in my direction like a large gun. They started to prepare me for my first treatment.

Switching on the monster, a light shined from it onto my neck where the tumor had been removed. This was just a test run, no radiation in the light. They focused the light so that it only showed on the part of my neck that needed treatment. I had to stay very still and not move after they had positioned the machine.

The nurse, using a large black waterproof marking pen, made an outline of the lighted area. I yelled out, "All I need is some feathers." I thought I looked like an Indian. Because the radiation had to be shined on the same place every time, those black marks stayed on my neck for weeks until the treatments were completed.

When it was time to let the machine run, the doctor and nurse went into another room, leaving me in the dark basement. I've never felt so alone in my life. It was extremely quiet.

Suddenly the machine came on and light shone on my neck, but I knew it wasn't just any light now. It was the radiation. I expected some kind of burning feeling on my neck, but there wasn't any. I had to sit completely still for the treatment and sitting there, waiting, seemed like it took forever. Finally, the light from the machine went off and the nurse came into the room and helped me back to my feet.

I went home and laid down for a nap to get my mind off the other treatments I still had ahead. There were more than I cared to have, but I trusted my doctor and followed his recommendations.

One good part of the treatments was the diet. I was told to eat a breakfast fit for four men to help to repair the skin tissues that were being affected by the radiation. My doctor was kind of heavy, so he just laughed when I told him I was putting on weight.

Even though the treatments were working, not all was OK. The repeated doses of radiation caused internal burning that closed up the artery in the right side of my neck. The doctors have never been able to fix or replace it. Now I have just one main artery in the left side of my neck — which only works at about 90% capacity — and the two small ones in the back. Fixing one illness caused problems elsewhere. Luckily this hasn't come back to get me yet. But because of this side effect, and for other reasons, I came to hate the radiation.

My fight with lymphoma had effects that went beyond the doctor's office. To deal with the difficulty of the treatment and my belief that I was going to die, I started drinking. I drank every day during the war, but never when I was on duty. I was a jolly good guy when I drank. When I got back from the war, I still drank some, but not very often. I was a weekend drinker. I'd have a beer sometimes, but I really liked Manhattans and Martinis.

After I was diagnosed with cancer, I figured that if I was going to go, I might as well go out numb. This got Marie upset. She didn't mind me drinking beers, but she didn't like the Manhattans and all that. But I'd have a couple of them and wouldn't feel the pain anymore and that's what I wanted. Soon enough I started drinking during the week, not just on the weekend. And I drank very heavily. I learned, though, that drinking wasn't the right way to deal with things.

Chapter 11
Dangerous Habits

While I was having my treatments, I tried to maintain as normal a life as possible, so I kept working and going to Rotary meetings and things like that. One night after a business event, I met some friends at a bar. Because they knew how much I liked the drink, they bought me Manhattans and I kept them buying. I don't know how many I had, but it was a bunch. Eventually I decided it was time to go home, and after I gave my name and address to the bartender he let me go.

At some point during my drive home, I lost all sense of what I was doing and where I was. Soon, I was struggling just to focus on the road. I looked in the rearview mirror and saw the flashing lights of a state trooper.

The lights told me I was in deep trouble, but I couldn't bring myself out of my drunkenness. I just couldn't get straight. If it got out that I'd been caught driving drunk, I would have to resign from all the clubs and business organizations to which I belonged. My reputation would be ruined.

I managed to pull over and my dear friend John Monko, who was also a competitor of mine, pulled up in front of me

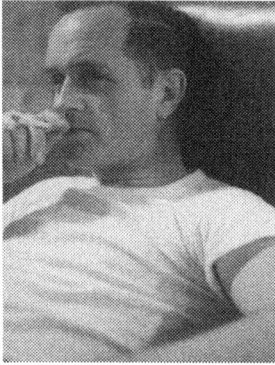

Drinking wasn't my only bad habit back then. I was a smoker, too.

before the trooper got out of his car. He'd been following me, I found out later, because he'd been worried that I'd had too much to drink. He walked over to my window and asked me how I was doing. I told him I was doing very badly. John told me to sit tight and went to speak to the trooper. He told the trooper about my situation, the cancer, my family. I don't know exactly what John said, but whatever it was, it worked.

The trooper came to the car with a ticket, and instructions to pull the car off the road and let John drive me home. It could have been much worse. He could have taken me to jail, but thanks to John he didn't. I'll always owe John for saving my reputation.

John came back and told me that he'd take care of me. I tried to get out of my car, but I blacked out a little. He drove me to a nearby McDonald's to get some coffee to sober me up. Coffee never worked that way for me, though. Instead, it kept me drunk and made me more awake to boot. We spent two hours drinking coffee and though I wasn't completely sober, I was solid enough to get my car and drive the short distance to my house.

The next morning, I went to work with a pounding head. As I came to the door of my office, I pulled out the ticket I'd gotten the night before. I was shocked to discover the reason the trooper pulled me over: I had been driving on the wrong side of the road.

Seeing that made me realize how badly I could have hurt my family. I thought of how I could have messed up another family. Realizing this, I quit serious drinking then and there. I did it on my own, without AA or any other help. I just plain stopped, and I haven't had a beer or drink of hard liquor in over twenty-five years. I have a glass of wine once in a while, but only ever one glass.

I wanted to write the trooper to thank him, to let him know that the trust he placed in me paid off. He'd given me a chance, given me a bit of trust, and it had worked out. I never did anything so stupid again. I wanted to let him know that something good came of it, because I'm sure police officers must give a lot of people the benefit of the doubt only to have it turn out badly.

Drinking wasn't my only bad habit back then. I was a smoker, too. At one point, I was burning through six packs of cigarettes a day. Imagine having to pay for that many packs today! I used to pay $0.38 a pack and I thought that was outrageous. I didn't smoke them all – I gave some away – but I smoked a lot of them. I was so hooked, in fact, that I used to wake up at night every hour on the hour for a smoke.

I had tried to quit more than once and every time I'd come back to it. My daughter Lynne used to tell me that the cigarettes made me stink, and though that made me want to quit, I just couldn't.

One night I was driving and as I reached to open my sixth pack of the day, I realized that I just wasn't enjoying smoking anymore. I quit then and there. I just flipped the cigarette out the window and said "I quit." I truly believe that I'd be dead now if I had continued to drink and smoke.

Quitting wasn't easy, though. I always wanted to smoke after I ate, but I didn't want to give in. So, when I felt the urge to smoke after eating, I would go downstairs to the basement where we had a table saw. I'd take a block of wood and cut a 90-degree angle in it. Once I'd done that, I'd smile, because the urge to smoke would have gone away. I'd distracted my mind and conquered my craving.

I had to do it that way because you can't just have one cigarette and anyone who's smoked for a while knows this. You think you're only going to have one, but you can't. My kids always used to ask me to quit, so I was doing it in part for them. They gave me extra willpower.

Looking back on it, I realize that being sick or going through hard times is no excuse to hurt yourself or someone else. You've got to hang in there. If you stay positive and don't give in, you'll pull through. I used to be so negative, but now when people ask me, "How are you doing?" my reply is, "Hanging in there with my short fingernails."

Chapter 12
Living On

After I got my diagnosis, I wanted to retire right away; I didn't want to retire when I would be very sick. Instead, I wanted to take some time to enjoy what I thought were going to be the last few years of my life. I wanted to see my country as best as I could in that time.

So we went to the Social Security office to find out if I could retire. I was in my 50s. At the time, I was having a hell of a hard time getting an insurance policy. The insurance companies thought I'd die before even making the first payment. And who could blame them? I thought I was a goner, too. But my brother Bobby worked on finding a policy for me.

Social Security said that I wasn't dying at the moment and I wasn't eligible for retirement yet. This put me at a real loss. I felt so helpless and so angry. There I was with cancer, with a wife at home and four grown children, who I wanted to see marry and have children of their own. I couldn't retire and I couldn't get insurance. I was in limbo and I didn't know what to do.

I thought about taking everyone to court because I wanted

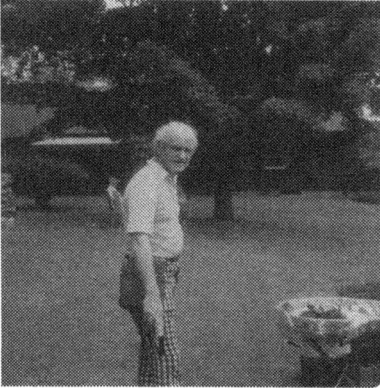

I couldn't retire and I couldn't get insurance. I was in limbo and I didn't know what to do.

some kind of answers. I wanted the judge to tell me if I was going to live or die. I felt I deserved some answers to my problems. Of course I couldn't take anyone to court – no one had done anything wrong. So I had to stay at work, stick with my treatments, and keep my fingers crossed.

Believe it or not, Bobby eventually found a company that would write a policy on me. A friend of his worked for the company. Still, they took me on one condition: I had to live three years before the policy came into full effect. Obviously that policy did come into effect.

The policy became active in 1984 when I turned 60, and even though A. Boilard Sons had its best five years ever as soon as I retired (no connection as far as I know!), I think I came out ahead of the game.

Chapter 13
More Lymphoma

When I didn't die from the lymphoma, I was disappointed. Not because I wanted to die, or thought I deserved to die, but because I had prepared myself. I'd set my mind to it, had gone to Confession, and I'd gotten everything ready. I was ready to die because I was expecting to and when I didn't it was quite an adjustment to make.

But I nearly got my chance again – a lot sooner than I would have liked.

Two years after I successfully completed the treatments for my first tumor, in March 1977, the doctor found a small lump on the left side of the neck. He thought it didn't belong there and should be taken out. So back on the table I went.

After testing, the tumor was found to be cancerous, so I knew I was in for more treatments. After what had happened to the arteries in my neck, I didn't want anymore radiation.

As an alternative, my new doctor, Doctor Flatow, suggested that I undergo chemotherapy treatments, which are administered intravenously. The treatments were to be done in his office, through my right hand. I was so relieved it wasn't

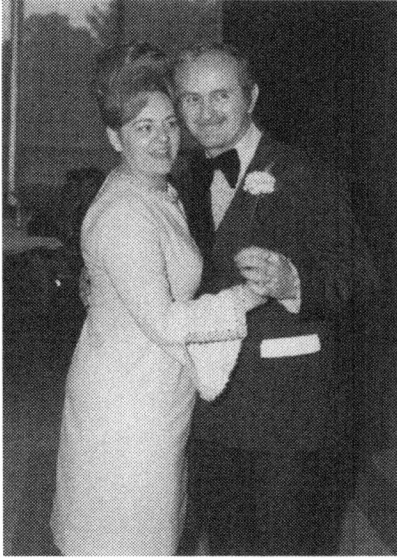

Two years after I successfully completed the treatments for my first tumor, in March 1977, the doctor found a small lump on the left side of the neck.

radiation that I quickly agreed to the plan.

I handled this treatment similarly to the radiation – I couldn't keep from joking with the girls in the office, but it was different, too – the place was well-lighted for a change. I waited in the office for the nurse to prepare the treatment. I was surprised when she wheeled out a set of large tubes filled to the top with this milky-looking stuff.

The doctor put the needle in my hand. That got more fun every time. I tell you, between all my treatments and stays in the hospital, I've had more pinpricks than a herd of porcupines.

It takes time to get all the treatment into the body. I'd often have to sit with the needle in my hand, letting the stuff drain into me, for hours. That wasn't much fun. It got made up for, though, by the light-headedness I ended up with. It was the kind of lightheadedness you get when you're on your third Manhattan. Of course, these treatments cost a lot more, and were a lot more serious, than a couple of cocktails!

I would joke with the doctor that he should tell the girls to watch out for me when I came out of the room. Of course, that was never more than a joke since after the treatments I'd have to sit in the car for about half an hour to get my head back on straight before I could drive. This went on for about eight weeks.

One of the greatest treats of chemotherapy was that about 24 hours after every treatment I'd throw up. It always seemed to come for me during the middle of a Rotary meeting. Luckily, the men there understood what I was going through.

After eight weeks of treatment – and throwing up – the doctor gave me the all clear. But that didn't last.

Because I'd had two cancers already, I was always on alert for trouble, as were the doctors when they checked me out. In 1986, I felt a swelling in my left armpit while in the shower washing under my arm. My heart dropped to my feet. I knew what it was. And I knew I was being knocked on my ass one more time. I wondered just how long I could take these knockdowns and keep getting up.

I went to the doctor with the problem. He told me what I already knew: it was another tumor. This time I had a friend of the family, Doctor Peck, take the tumor out.

I got a milder chemo treatment this time and it worked. I haven't gotten lymphoma again, but this wasn't my last fight with cancer. Not by a long shot.

Chapter 14
Belief

I hope there's a God. But I don't know about heaven — I figure it would be pretty crowded up there with all the good people. Still, I'd like to believe that there is a heaven.

I don't think there's anything wrong with believing in God. I think it's a useful thing. It gives me someone to talk to.

Since I was brought up Catholic, I believe that God is in you, in each of us. So when I talk to myself, when I pray, I'm actually talking to God and the answers I get are from God.

I've talked to God my whole life. My parents raised us to be good Roman Catholics, so we went to church every Sunday and holiday. No matter what the weather was, we all walked to mass down on Main St. in Indian Orchard. In those days, different churches held their masses in different languages. If you were Catholic in Indian Orchard you could choose from masses said in Polish, Italian, or French. There were Irish Catholic churches, too, and those masses were in English. We went to the French church. I also liked going to the Polish church on Parker St., just around the corner from our house. Whenever I went there, though, I always seemed to be late, which in those days meant all the pews were full and you had

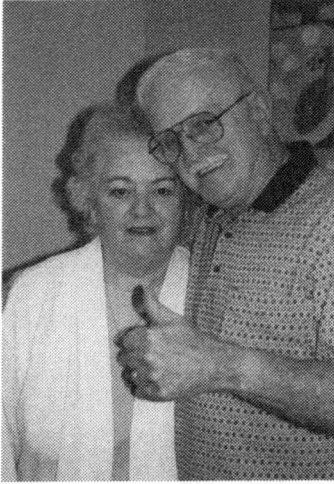

Instead, the Lord and I have some blow-by-blow talks. I say, "Hey Lord, I got enough goddamned trouble now. You want me, take me!"

to stand in the back with the other latecomers.

My doctors have told me that they always thank God that people believe in a heaven. That belief makes it easier for people to die peacefully, they say. When people believe in an afterlife, when they believe in resurrection, they're able to die more easily.

Though I've had some pretty low moments, I never sit there and wait to die. Instead, the Lord and I have some blow-by-blow talks. I say, "Hey Lord, I got enough goddamned trouble now. You want me, take me!"

I wait a second and when I'm still there, I smile and say, "OK, I'm sorry."

Besides these talks, I've prayed to God for many things: money or a pretty girl, health for loved ones. Not all my prayers got answered, but the important ones did. I was blessed with a beautiful home, a beautiful girl to call my wife and to share my life with, and four wonderful children.

So to me there is a God. It's somebody who's in you, who you talk to yourself, who gives you answers. You just hope you get the right answers!

Chapter 15
Try Talking About It
(even if no one lets you)

During my recovery from lymphoma, Doctor Flatow asked me if I would be interested in joining a therapy group for people with cancer. I resisted the idea at first: I didn't think there was anything I could do to help other folks and I didn't see how they could help me. But because of my outlook on life and the way I accepted the disease, Doctor Flatow thought I might help some of them. So I agreed to go.

A group of about 10 of us met at the YMCA in Springfield. Some were old and some were very young. These were the hardest for me to accept. There was even a young woman who had just given birth to a child and now she had cancer. It broke my heart to hear her talk about her new baby one minute and the next about the sickness that might mean her child would grow up without her mom. I wondered what God was thinking letting this beautiful young mother have cancer. I never figured it out.

Though Doctor Flatow had convinced me to join the group because he thought I might have something valuable to share, I hardly got the chance. Everyone else talked and talked

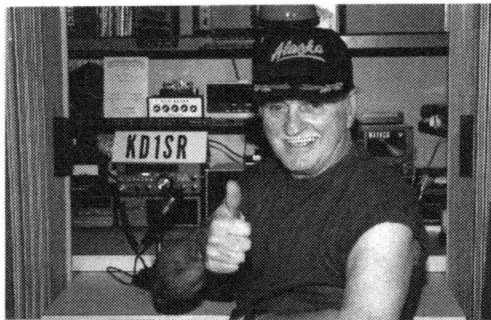

But believe me when I tell you that hearing a doctor say that there are no signs of cancer in you feels like winning the Super Bowl, or the World Series.

and I barely got a word in edgewise. Everyone talked about their take on the disease. The older folks said they were going to beat it and the young asked "why me?" I never said either of these things. I never felt that I would beat cancer, but just wanted to live the life God gave me.

It was sad to see how desperate some people got in the face of cancer. One of the older men in the group who said he was going to lick it was so desperate that he went to Canada for a quack treatment. The treatment went like this: He would pour this jelly over his body and let it dry. Then he'd pull it off in one big sheet and hanging from the sheet were supposed to be these cancer "worms", taken out of his body. The poor man was so desperate that he was willing to try anything that might help, even something that didn't make sense. And of course there are folks out there who know this and try to take advantage of people.

This scam didn't help and that man died.

I went to a couple more therapy classes before I stopped. I couldn't take it anymore, especially the fact that I never got a chance to talk.

The same problem would crop up at work. I had many wonderful customers and they knew I had a serious illness, so they would come to me and say how sorry they were to hear that I had cancer. I always thanked them, but tried to avoid talking about it more than that. It seemed that when I did talk about it the other person would bring up a story about how they were feeling about their problems, as if their attempts to make me feel better included telling me that others were worse off. I knew then, just as I know now, that that's true, but it didn't help. So I tried not to talk about it unless someone was really interested in finding out how I was doing.

After I left the group I went back to my way of thinking: I'll never beat it. Even though I seem to be OK now and there's no active cancer in my body today, I believe it could pop up again at any time.

But believe me when I tell you that hearing a doctor say that there are no signs of cancer in you feels like winning the Super Bowl, or the World Series, or getting the chance to go to bed with Marilyn Monroe. Just to sleep, of course, but still.

Chapter 16
Just Keep Going

You see some people get sick and they don't do anything but spend all their time being sick. It becomes who they are. And they spend hours wondering, "What did I do? Why me?"

Well, not me. During the years that I battled cancer, I tried to forget about it and to live what life God had left for me. What choice did I have?

After the first tumor was removed, I gave myself at most five years to live. Well, before I knew it, I was in my sixth year and disappointed that I hadn't died.

Once that passed, though, I started to get back on track, feeling positive about having a future. I got checked twice a year and prayed a lot. I never thought I'd lick cancer; I just accepted it and went on with life.

My family was very supportive, especially Marie. I remember her looking at me as I lay sick in bed and I could see in her eyes that she would have done anything I needed to help me. She would have given me her heart if it would have helped.

There were many tough moments.

One day in the hospital during my first lymphoma-related

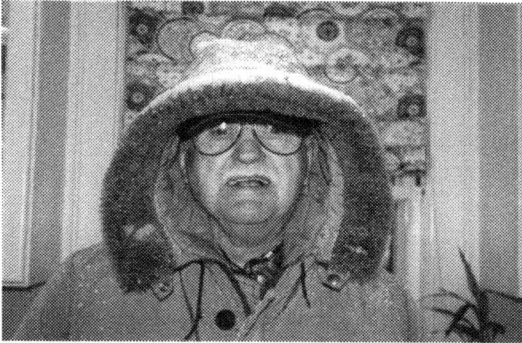

During the years that I battled cancer, I tried to forget about it and to live what life God had left for me. What choice did I have?

stay, I hit maybe the lowest point of my life. I was lying in bed, feeling awful, being quiet. I didn't want to do anything. I didn't want to talk, to eat, to get up. I think I was getting ready to die.

One of the nurses brought in a plate of food, covered with a silver top, and a cup of coffee. I didn't want to have it, but the nurse asked me to sit up and drink some of the coffee. Then she left.

I sat up to have the coffee. The tray of food was resting on my bed. I got curious about what was under the lid, and after lifting it discovered that it was my favorite food: shepherd's pie.

I put the cover back on the food and put my head in my hands and then let it fall to my chin. I started to cry and it seemed like time just slowed down. I could hear the teardrops falling onto the metal plate cover, making big "ploom, ploom" noises, like slow motion in the movies.

The world was narrowing down to a point, getting smaller and smaller. I know now that I was leaving the world. I was mentally checking out.

The next thing I knew, the doctor was on the bed, slapping me in the face.

"What's the matter with you?" he said. "You're going to

get to go home."

That scared me. I worried that maybe I would never have been able to come out of it. But luckily I never had to find out. I never got that bad again.

While trying to recover, I tried to dress the best I could. That might not seem important, but to me it was. When people get diagnoses of cancer and things like that, they take it hard. A lot of them go home and get in bed and let themselves go to hell. They don't get out of bed, don't wash or dress, they do nothing for months and then they just die. I never wanted to be like that. Marie handled that job for me and did wonderfully making sure I was well dressed and looking good to others. Looking good and not like a mess helped me feel good and keep a positive attitude. It can be hard to keep up one's appearance when battling cancer or other problems, but I think it helps.

This is part of why I wanted to write this book. I wanted to show people that there are other ways to live with these illnesses, productive ways.

Now I keep going because I have passion for so many subjects. I don't want to miss the chance to learn more about them, to better my skills, to do new things. I'm always looking far ahead of whatever I'm doing. With one of my hobbies, photography, I'm always looking at new cameras to buy and saving up for them. Then, when I've got them, I know that I've got to learn how to use them and take the best advantage of what they can do.

On the personal side, I have two new great-granddaughters and a great-grandson who I'm looking forward to seeing more. The promise of seeing them keeps me going, too. I also have eight step-great-grandchildren who give me great joy.

The way I see it, if you make enough plans, you'll be too busy to stop!

Chapter 17
Keep Busy, Keep Learning

Whether you're healthy or sick, life is best when you keep your mind active and your hands busy. This is especially true when you're sick, because it'll keep your mind off your troubles.

I've got a few hobbies that have kept me growing and challenged over the years.

One of them is art, which I've always enjoyed. I drew pictures and took photos when I was a boy and I kept it up during the war. I used to decorate my letters to Marie with little icons – I was using them decades before anyone put them in the computer!

I especially enjoy making drawings with pen and ink and filling them in and finishing them up with watercolors.

I like to make drawings for children. I often do my version of Holly Hobby for girls or a sports or karate caricature or something like that for boys.

I also used to make Christmas cards by hand. Once I got a computer, I started making them that way. Now I only have to make one card and can scan it into the computer – no more making each one by hand like in the past. I've done two years

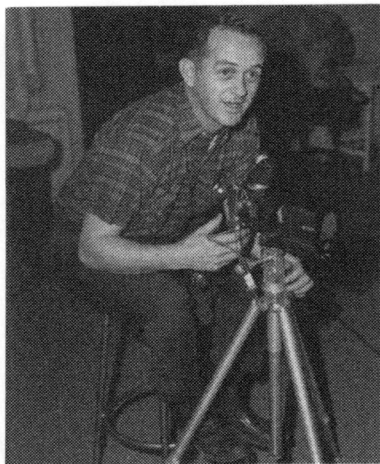

One year Marie bought me an Argus C3 for Christmas, which was a big step up for me. Later we even put an addition on the house to allow me to have a photo studio.

worth of cards in advance and they're saved in the computer. That way, even if I die, people will still get Christmas cards from me for a few years!

Along with drawing, I've taken photographs for many years.

I got started as a photographer when I was a boy of 11 or so and bought a camera for $0.25 at a store. All I had was the camera, though. I didn't have a dark room or a way to develop the pictures. Luckily one of my friends had the whole set up and he showed me how. Once I learned about the development process, I got some chemicals and spent hours as a boy developing photos and negatives in bowls in my closet.

After I returned from the war I got ahold of a Leica camera, which is a pretty fancy item. I took a few photos with it and entered some of them into local photo club contests. None of those photos won anything, but I liked the exposure and the process and kept going with it.

I took pictures of children, especially our kids, in all sorts of funny poses. I also took a lot of nature photos – birds, bears, big cats. I love my nature photos and am very proud of them.

I used to take a lot of photos of sunrises and sunsets. In the early days of making them, though, they seemed to be missing something. A friend of mine looked at them and told me I needed to add silhouettes to them. Every good sunrise or sunset photo needs a silhouette, he said. But where was I going to find things to silhouette in the photos?

Instead of getting real, live pictures, I worked out a way to fake them a bit. I cut out some silhouettes of ducks from a hunting magazine and projected them against a wall. Then I projected one of my sunsets onto the same wall so that my duck silhouettes were laid over the sunset photo. With the picture created on the wall, I took a roll or two of the new pictures.

I liked how they came out very well and entered them into some local contests. I even won some ribbons! I didn't tell anyone at the contests about how I made the pictures, but I did tell my friend. He said it was fine, that it didn't matter how the picture was made, but whether or not you liked the end result. I definitely liked the end result.

As I got more involved in photography, I got better equipment. One year Marie bought me an Argus C3 for Christmas, which was a big step up for me. Later we even put an addition on the house to allow me to have a photo studio. The addition was 24 x 24 feet and there was about an eight-foot room I used as a studio and changing area where I shot pictures of children and models.

My hobby led me to join the Springfield Camera Club and the New England Camera Council. I attended the New England Camera Council's annual meeting at UMass Amherst for years. We'd take over the campus, live in the dorms,

Chapter 17: Keep Busy, Keep Learning

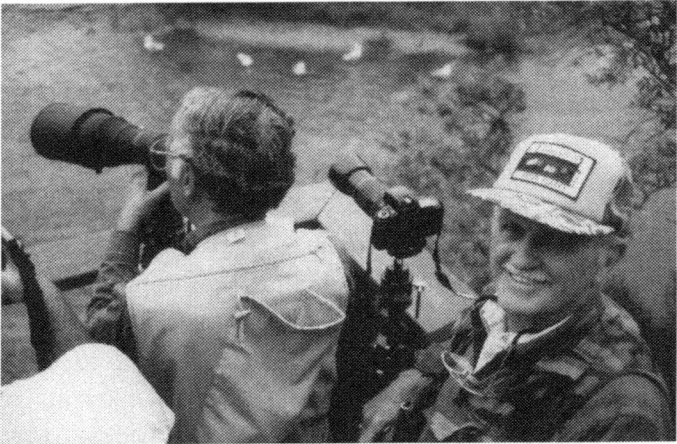

Here I am in Alaska, with my best buddy Harry, photographing bears.

give lectures, attend meetings, between 1,200 and 1,600 of us. As I became more involved, I started to give lectures on photographing children and nature. These lectures took me around the country – to California, New York, Canada – which was great. Along with helping me pursue something I loved, both groups were great for making new friends.

I think making art is a wonderful hobby for all sorts of people. If you have an interest, develop it. If you can draw, do it, even if you have to start out copying others. You'll learn from that. If you can't draw, pick up a camera. It doesn't have to be those two things, really. Just making any kind of art is good for you.

I have other hobbies, too, like ham radio. I've used my radio to talk to people all over the world, as far away as Germany, I've talked to college professors, and I talk to my nephew almost every day using the radio.

My dad was a photographer, too, but he didn't take still photos – he took movies. He'd always take movies of things the family did; holidays, weddings, religious events, family picnics, and gatherings.

When dad died I inherited all his cameras and film. When we counted up all the 8mm and 16mm film, it was 55,000 feet of film!

I watched a lot of the film and found that dad had taken some terrific movies of us. I decided to do something with the movies for the family. So, one year while I was on vacation, I watched the film and spliced some segments together to make a longer movie about the family. By this time we had a video camera, too. So I projected the film onto the wall and played some tapes in the background while I videotaped the projection. It was low tech, but I was able to make a whole movie, including a soundtrack, that way!

I made copies of the movie and gave the VHS tapes to everyone in the family. Recently my daughter Michelle put the movie on DVD so it will last forever.

When the doctors tell you you've got cancer or another serious problem, it knocks you on your ass. You spend a few days lying around, feeling bad, but then you've got a choice: you are either going to keep on feeling bad until you die or you get up and say I've got to keep going, so I'm going to do what I love. Having art in my life, and being able to make other people happy with it, has always helped me choose the second option.

Chapter 18
Battling Kidney Stones

If you're looking for pain – though I don't know why you would be – kidney stones will supply it for you. I've had two bouts with them and I'm hoping not to see a third. I've been run over by a truck and survived surgeries and chemotherapy, but they were nothing compared to the pain of kidney stones.

A kidney stone, for those who don't know, is a hard mass that develops in the kidneys when something goes wrong with the chemicals in your urine. Many times these little stones will pass right out of the body when you pee, but when they don't, whoa boy! That's when the pain starts up. And it can be a whopper, let me tell you.

The first time I got kidney stones was in 1980. It was a Friday. I woke up to go to work and went to the bathroom for a morning pee. But nothing came out. Well, that's pretty strange, I thought. What the hell's going on? Nothing hurt, though, so I went to work.

I had a Rotary meeting that night and my back was giving me some pain, so I didn't eat anything. By the time the meeting was done, the pain was so bad that I called Marie and had her take me to the hospital. We were supposed to be flying to

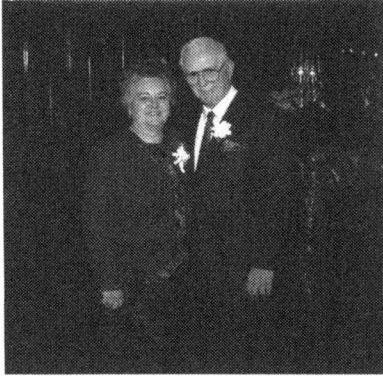

We were supposed to be flying to Atlantic City for a vacation the next day. Needless to say, we didn't make it.

Atlantic City for a vacation the next day. Needless to say, we didn't make it.

In the hospital, they had me drink some liquid that made it easier for them to see inside me. Then they laid me down on the X-ray table and the doctor had a look.

"You're not having any pain now, are you?" he asked.

I told him he was right and he replied that he couldn't find the kidney stone. He'd seen it for a minute, but then it disappeared. The pain disappeared, too, so that was OK with me. He sent me home.

Later, I was going to the bathroom. All of a sudden the urine stopped and there was a pain so bad that I nearly passed out. I fell forward and had to prop myself against the wall to keep from going all the way down. Then I heard "crunk crunk crunk" and the urine started again. I looked into the toilet and there were the missing kidney stones! They were about a quarter inch in diameter. Looking at those things made me think that we're all oysters, just making pearls.

Later in my life, I had another attack. I went to the hospital again, and again they couldn't find the thing. They sent me home and though I don't remember passing it, I must have, because it's sure not in there now!

Chapter 19
My First Heart Attack

I t was August 1989 and it was very hot. I was loading my antenna beam onto the roof of the car. As I walked back and forth getting rope and tying the antenna, I started to sweat. Soon, the sweat was pouring off me. I had to tie my hankie to my forehead to keep the sweat out of my eyes. I suddenly got very weak. I began to stagger as I walked. I decided I needed a rest and that I was going to go in the house, lie down and take a couple of Tylenol. Luckily I didn't get that far. I later learned this would have been the worst thing I could have done.

I began to talk to myself, but not very loud because I didn't want folks to hear me and think I was nuts.

"You feel lousy, Chick, right? Think you should go to the hospital? Best thing I can think of to do. Okay, go get Marie and have her take you."

Marie was soon at the wheel and with about eight miles to the hospital I started to get pain in my shoulders. The pain was so bad I didn't know where to put myself. I told Marie to hurry up. Her reply was, "I can't fly over the big trucks." At this point I was still thinking that I just had a severe case of

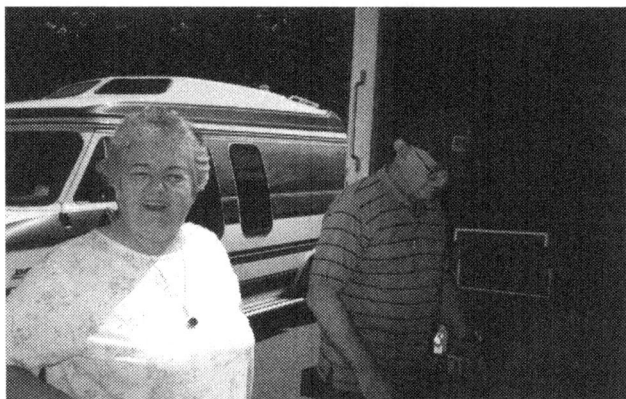

heat stroke.

When we got to the emergency room at Mercy Hospital in Springfield, I had just about had it. A nurse and a police officer came running out pushing a wheelchair and opened the car door. They asked if I could get out of the car and into the wheelchair. "Piece of cake," I replied and started to get up. But I couldn't. I couldn't move at all. They had to drag me out of the car.

I was rushed into an exam room and six people picked me up and put me on a table. With one person at each arm they put in intravenous lines. A doctor checked my heart and told me I was having a heart attack. I looked at her, asking with my eyes, "What do you want me to do?" She asked who my doctor was and I managed to tell her it was Dr. Flatow, whose office was just two blocks away.

Dr. Flatow was there in a flash, with a heart specialist named Dr. Carney.

"How long ago did you start having the pain?" they asked.

"Less then an hour ago," was my answer. The doctors were able to use what I think was a new medication for keeping my heart from getting damaged. One shot of it cost about $2,600.00.

I was then taken to the ICU for the nurses to observe how I was doing. I remember being knocked out. Man, I was sleeping very soundly. When I woke up, I thought I was in a spaceship. It was dark and the doctors and nurses were all in green clothes. There was lots of equipment with blinking lights and monitors showing all types of pictures. I could have been in outer space. I got scared. It took a few minutes, but I realized that I was in the hospital ICU, so I settled down.

I recovered from this heart attack and regained my strength. I got myself through the way I always do: I sang myself songs to keep my spirits up and to keep myself company and I joked with the nurses. Lifting the spirits of others always helps to lift ones' own, I find.

Chapter 20
How My Daughter Tried to Kill Me

When I tell the story of my second heart attack, I like to say that it was a result of my daughter Michelle trying to kill me. It's not true, of course, and she feels badly about it, but I like to tease. That's my sense of humor!

In 1996, Marie and I celebrated our 50th anniversary. Michelle and her husband Bob offered to take us anywhere in the world. I wanted to go to Europe and see the site of D-Day and other famous World War II battles. We spent 10 days visiting and had a wonderful vacation touring Belgium, the Netherlands, Germany, and France.

When we were in France we rented a car and drove around the countryside and had an enjoyable time. When we were in Paris we saw the Eiffel Tower, of course, and then went to the Arc De Triomphe. On the day we visited, the elevator wasn't working, but I was feeling strong so I encouraged Michelle to go with me and we got in line to go inside.

While we were waiting, one of the guards came up to me.

"It's 284 steps, sir," he kept saying (though some say it's more, some say less). "Are you sure you want to walk?"

Chapter 20: How My Daughter Tried to Kill Me

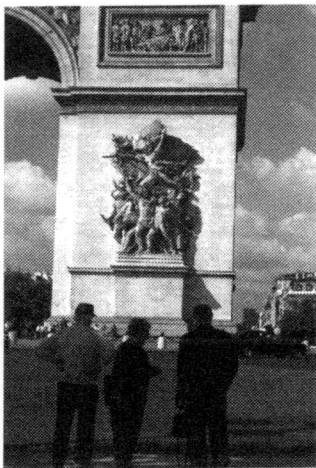

While we were waiting, one of the guards came up to me. "It's 284 steps, sir," he kept saying. "Are you sure you want to walk?"

I told him I was tough and he let me go.

Finally Michelle and I got inside and we started to climb the stairs. The staircase in the Arc is narrow and winding, only wide enough for a single-file line heading up. We kept up a good pace with the line, but about halfway up, I started to feel pretty pooped and had to take a break. Because the line was single file, everyone behind us had to stop too. It was a good thing that I didn't have a heart attack then — it would have taken forever to get me out.

After I'd had my rest, we started walking again and eventually made it to the top. We waited at the top for a while, so I could catch my breath. Once I'd caught it, we went back down. Going down was a lot easier!

A few days after we returned home I was helping Marie bring in some shopping bags. It was a very warm day on Cape Cod and I began to feel the same way I did when I had my first heart attack. I was weak and sweating, but this time the pain came early. I sat down and told Marie that I was not fooling around and that she should call 911 right away.

An ambulance arrived quickly. They gave me oxygen and a shot to keep me quiet and off we went to Hyannis Hospital.

As we were backing up to the hospital ramp I passed out. Because I was out, I don't know what happened, but I was told that after three hours the doctors at Hyannis Hospital couldn't get me stabilized, so they sent me to Brigham and Women's Hospital in Boston. I awoke briefly on the ride to Boston, but again, as they backed the ambulance up to the hospital ramp, I passed out.

It was at Brigham and Women's that I finally woke up. They were saying they couldn't open the veins. We've got to do something about this, they told me.

Chapter 21
Heart Bypass Surgery

The doctors at Brigham and Women's knew that the blood vessels near my heart were too constricted to let the blood flow properly, so they took some immediate action – an angioplasty. They inserted a small plastic ball with a hole in it into a blood vessel near my heart. With the ball keeping the vessel open and the blood pumping through the hole, I was set for a little while.

But as soon as this was done, they started prepping me for a more serious, but also more useful, surgery – a heart bypass.

About a month after I was released from the hospital for my angioplasty, Michelle and Marie drove me back to Brigham and Women's for the bypass. After getting checked in and tested, the doctors and nurses prepped me for the surgery. When the time came to take me for the operation, I was wheeled through the hospital on a bed. I counted the ceiling tiles as they passed overhead, something I've always done on my way to surgery. The last thing I remember is a large group of doctors and nurses being there to greet me in the operating room.

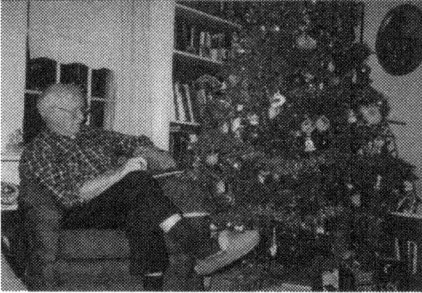

Marie and I are normally in Florida at Christmas, so this was our first white Christmas in many years.

The next thing I remember is waking up in the ICU with Marie, Michelle, Lynne, and Chris. They were the first things I saw when I opened my eyes. What a wonderful sight!

I, on the other hand, wasn't such a pretty sight. I had all sorts of tubes and connections sticking in and out of me.

I stayed in bed for a while, recovering and letting the doctors and nurses take care of me. I did make one mistake during the stay, though. When the nurses would come by to check on me and my pain, they'd always ask where the pain landed on a scale of one to ten. Now, I didn't know which end of that scale was which, so I always told them 10!

After I did this a few times, I started to understand why people would get after pain pills. I'd take the pills the nurses gave me for pain I didn't actually have and soon enough the wallpaper would be running down the walls like water. The only things that didn't move were the picture, light switch, and charts.

I tried to stay away from the pain pills after that.

Part of my recovery was checking the capacity of my lungs and strength of my stitches. In order to do this, the doctors would have me cough a number of times. This hurt a great deal. To help deal with the pain, the doctors suggested I hug a pillow when I coughed. Sometimes it took two pillows for me to help keep the pain down.

Michelle noticed the pillows and went out and bought me a very large stuffed gray wolf that I could hug when the pain got too bad. It did the job. Sometimes folks passing my room would stop back and check to see if it was a real wolf, believe it or not.

Soon enough I was released from the hospital. Marie and I went to stay at Michelle and Bob's home in Worcester for my recuperation. The holidays were coming and so we stayed through Christmas, even helping them pick out a Christmas tree. Marie and I are normally in Florida at Christmas, so this was our first white Christmas in many years.

Right after the holidays, we boarded a plane for Florida and headed home. The operation had been a great success.

Chapter 22
Love

Surviving my illnesses gave me an opportunity: to love my family and friends as much and as hard as I can. Since I never thought I was going to make it a long time anyway, I decided I had nothing to lose in telling everyone how I felt.

I want to be the very best friend I can be and to have the very best of friends. I want my family to know that I love them and to feel my love for them. It truly helps to have loving family and friends to cheer you on, so I want to give some of that love back.

I go out of my way to tell them "I love you." I hug them, I kiss them, and I say "I love you very much." I think it's important to tell them, because it costs you nothing and it means so much to people.

I also love people that I don't know, women and men, young and old. I am quick to say hello to a pretty girl – though I always stop myself from declaring love! Some may think that I'm a little too bold but I try to keep my sense of humor and be friendly. I think that old folks are great, but I especially

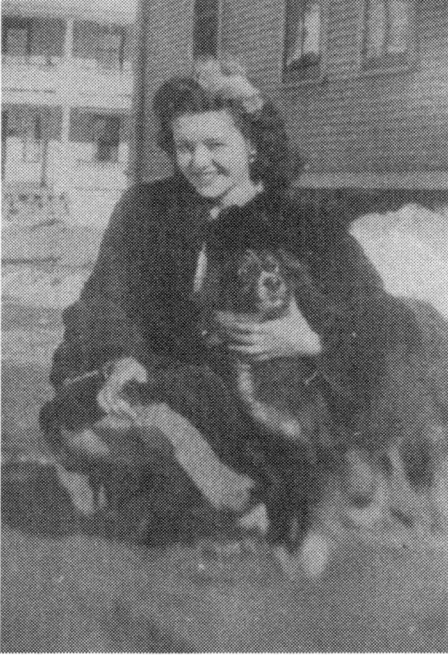

Surviving my illnesses gave me an opportunity: to love my family and friends as much and as hard as I can.

love children. I keep a list of about thirty names of children and people who I think are young at heart and try to stay in touch with them regularly. I send many of them my drawings and Christmas cards.

Chapter 23
Surviving Prostate Cancer

During a routine visit, my doctor in Florida checked my PSA level, which is what they look at to make sure you don't have prostate cancer. Because of my medical history, the reading he got concerned him. I thought that it wasn't too bad but I asked him what he suggested. He suggested radiation because taking my prostate out was too big an operation with my bad heart.

I headed north to see what my doctors up there would suggest. They thought maybe the reading was OK, but decided to go along with my doctor in Florida. At first they wanted to do a surgery that would have cut my groin and inner legs open in a huge flap. Needless to say that option didn't interest me too much! I was pretty happy to take the radiation this time.

It was decided that I would have radiation treatments five days a week for four or five weeks. I'd have to go to the hospital every day to get the treatments, so I needed to pick a regular hospital to go to. We were living in Wellfleet on Cape Cod then and the closest hospital to us was Hyannis Hospital, 30 miles from our place. That was closer than going to Boston, which was my other option, but I still ended up putting 2,400

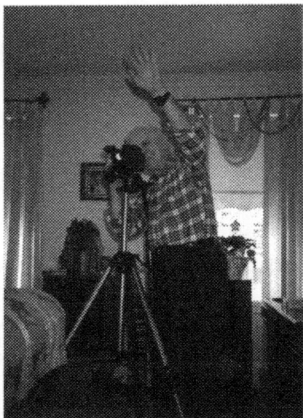

I still ended up putting 2,400 miles on the car in only one month!

miles on the car in only one month!

The treatments weren't too bad. But I hated radiation after what it did to the artery in my neck. And I was right to feel that way.

This illness also showed me the value of getting good supplemental insurance. We had MediCare, but having supplemental insurance saved us a bundle. Marie calculated once that it probably saved us hundreds of thousands of dollars over the years. Good thing we had it. Without it, we could have been ruined.

Chapter 24
Cancer, Again

By 1999, Marie and I were enjoying our retirement in Florida. But the smooth sailing didn't last. I started to pass blood in my urine. That would worry anybody, but it worried me more because there was so much of it. I looked at it and said to myself, "well, this is it. We've all got to go sometime and this must be my time."

I called the doctor immediately and they quickly brought me in for an examination. The exam was done by putting a tube up through the urinary tract to get a good look at the inside of my bladder – and you men know what this means and just how much fun it is. The procedure wasn't too awful, but after that tube came out, it did take three days for my eyes to uncross.

The results of the test were serious: The doctor found two tumors. With all the blood, though, that wasn't such a big surprise. The surprise was that the tumors were bleeding so early. Normally, the doctor told me, that kind of tumor doesn't bleed so early in its growth. It turned out that the blood thinners I was taking for my heart contributed to the early bleeding. A treatment I was taking for one thing helped

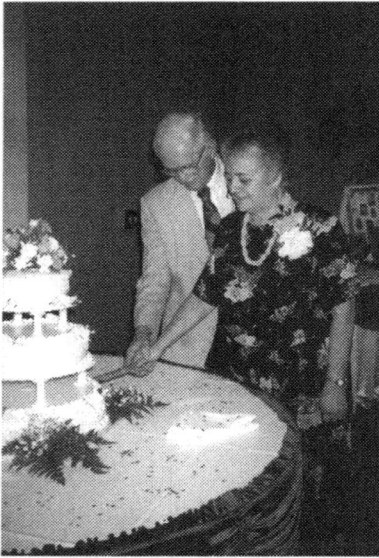

Marie and I celebrating our 50th anniversary in 1996. By this time we were happily retired and living in Florida.

me discover another in time to get it cured. Score one for me and all my illnesses.

I had to go to the hospital to have the tumors taken out. That wasn't so tough. But then I had to have treatments, called BCG. Not only was that trickier, I really got to hate those treatments. And they were the only ones available to me — the damage from the radiation years before kept me from having other types of treatments.

I learned that BCG is one of the most common ways to treat bladder cancer. It's mixed into a solution and then put directly in the bladder to help the body's natural defenses fight the cancer.

Once a week for six weeks I would drive to the doctor's office in Springfield for a treatment. The doctor would put the contents of a little bottle (at a cost of $100.00 per bottle) the size of a golf ball into my bladder, through a catheter in the urinary tract.

That was uncomfortable of course (there was a lot of eye-crossing for me in those days), but the real hard part was that I was supposed to hold the BCG in my bladder for two hours. After the BCG was in there, I was supposed to roll around to make sure that it washed over all sides of my bladder for the most effective treatment.

The BCG seemed to do the trick and my three-month check-up found my bladder clear of cancer.

I was healthy for a year. No bleeding, no tumors, good health. But then the bleeding started again. My spirits hit the floor when the doctor told me there were two more tumors growing and I would have to have them removed and go through the BCG treatments again.

My sadness turned to anger and I was ready to give up — again. It took me about three days to talk myself out of this. I did that by reminding myself how blessed I was in love and family and friends. Then I began to cheer up. The anger went away and was replaced by fear. I really didn't want to die and so I took out the big guns – my sense of humor. I found every opportunity to tell jokes and poke fun at myself and my situation. This not only helped me get through, but seemed to help everyone around me, too.

When the doctors determined that it was bladder cancer again, I had another surgery. I remember a funny moment from after the surgery. Lynne had come to visit me in the hospital and Michelle had called us on the phone to see how I was doing.

I told her that they were showing me movies. She asked what kind.

"They're showing me porno movies," I told her. "To make sure everything's still working!"

I then handed the phone to Lynne. Michelle asked Lynne about the tumor and she replied that it was small.

From the background, I called out to Michelle, "She's talking about the tumor!"

For the follow-up treatment, my doctor in Springfield suggested I try a new therapy, a combination of BCG and Interferon. I was cautious, but agreed. After each treatment, Marie would drive me to our daughter Lynne's home in Belchertown, Ma., so I could roll the mixture around my bladder as instructed.

Keeping it in is really hard, remember, so when I would get to Lynne's after the 20-mile car ride, I was always ready to pee. Extremely ready. My eyes would nearly be turning yellow. The doctor instructed me to have a small bottle of bleach to pour over the urine that was in the toilet.

Sounds simple, right? Well it wasn't that easy. I always had to go but nothing would come out. The pain of needing to and not being able was awful. Given enough time, though, a little bit would come out and I'd pour the beach over it, leave it there for fifteen minutes, and flush.

After one particular treatment I just couldn't go, no matter how long I waited. The pain was so bad that Lynne's husband John drove me to the emergency room around midnight. I hung around in a wheelchair for about an hour before they brought me to a room and put in a catheter.

I said to the nurse, "Watch out, here comes Old Faithful!"

It was so wonderful to feel the urine flow out through that tube; I now know how it will feel to go to heaven.

Soon enough the doctor did another check up and found no cancer and it's been three years since there was any cancer in my bladder. When he told me the good news, I tried to hug him, but he wouldn't let me.

I loved my two doctors, the one in Florida and the one in Massachusetts. The one in Springfield was always serious — he was seeing a lot of people that he just couldn't save. But I was his bright star: no matter what happened, I just kept coming back to him.

One thing I learned from all my battles with cancer: do what the doctor says. I truly believe that it is because of their determination and dedication that I am still here.

Chapter 25
Fighting Off a Bat Attack

When spring comes around each year, we leave Florida and head north to be with the family. Our daughters and son always make sure we have a fine time.

Michelle has a very large home in Worcester. She and her husband, Bob, fixed up a wonderful room for us — twin beds, cable TV, red walls, and a desk — where we stay for most of the summer.

One summer night while Marie and I were watching TV on the big Sony in the living room, I saw a dark object fly by my head. I didn't get a good look at it, but I got another chance as it quickly came our way again.

I thought it was a bird or a bat and I decided to see if I could find something to catch it with. Remember, I've hunted wild animals. It slowed down a bit and I saw that it was a bat. We couldn't figure out how it got into the house.

I tried to catch it, but nothing that Michelle or Marie gave me was good enough to get it out of the air, so instead I decided to bide my time and wait until it landed somewhere. Then I'd make my move.

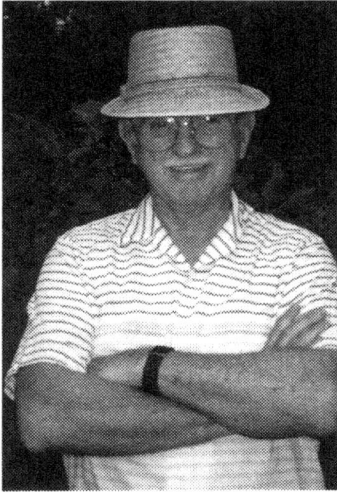

I wore a pair of heavy-duty work gloves and not much more protection.

After following it around the house for a while, it finally landed on the drapes in the second floor hallway. I approached it cautiously and wrapped my hand around it, with the drapes between the bat and my hand. The bat wasn't too happy to have been caught and let me know by nipping my hand while I was trying to get the thing untangled from the drapes.

I wanted to get it outside, but didn't want to get bitten again, so I grabbed it by the wing tips to try to keep its mouth away from my hand. That didn't work. It just turned around and bit me again, this time drawing blood.

You never know what kinds of diseases bats might be carrying, so we decided that I should get to the hospital. Michelle and Marie took me to the emergency room at Memorial Hospital in Worcester.

I was the hit of the emergency room. The Batman, they called me! The doctor looked me over and told me I'd need some rabies shots. I had seven shots the first night and an additional shot each week for the next six weeks. I could have saved myself all that trouble if I'd brought the bat into the hospital where they could have tested it for rabies, but since I hadn't, they had to be safe and give me all those shots.

As usual, I tried to lighten the mood with jokes. When the nurses came in to see where the bat had bitten me, I told them that they couldn't see the bite because it was on my penis. I told them, too, that I was considering charging for the privilege. Everyone got a kick out of that.

I was still getting my shots from the first encounter with the bat when another one showed up in the house.

This time I was ready.

As the bat flew downstairs Michelle and Marie went to get some protective equipment. Michelle had a very large hat on, a scarf around her neck, and a tennis racket in her hand. Marie had on about the same outfit. They looked like low-tech Ghostbusters.

On the other hand, I wore a pair of heavy-duty work gloves and not much more protection. This time the bat landed in the third-floor drapes and up I went. I got a gloved hand around the bat and brought it outside, where I hit it with a rock a few times. I don't know if I killed it, though, because I left it out there and in the morning it was gone.

Because two bats had been in the house in a week, Michelle and Bob were worried that there might be bats in the attic or a hole somewhere that they were getting in through. Michelle hired a man who specialized in dealing with bats to come over and check it out. When he heard about how I handled them, he offered me a job. He said he could use a guy like me for his team! I didn't accept, though — I was enjoying my retirement.

Chapter 26
My Trip to La La Land

Two-Thousand Four was one of the toughest years I've ever seen. If my life up to that point could have been all rolled together and baked into a cake, 2004 would have been the frosting.

I barely remember any of that year, in fact. I know bits and pieces, but I have to rely on other people to tell me what happened. It was that kind of year.

It started, like a lot of things do for a lot of older people, with a fall. I was walking behind Marie up the front steps of Michelle and Bob's house when I lost my balance and started to fall. I twisted my body around to keep from knocking my head against the concrete steps. I twisted one of my legs, too. I succeeded in my goal: I missed the steps and landed in the grass. I felt OK at the time, but I had no idea what was in store for me.

The next day I had some pain in the leg I'd twisted, so I went to see the doctor. He ordered some X-rays of my hip and knee, but they didn't show anything.

Everything seemed OK, but when I came downstairs for breakfast the next day, I collapsed in the kitchen. Marie tried

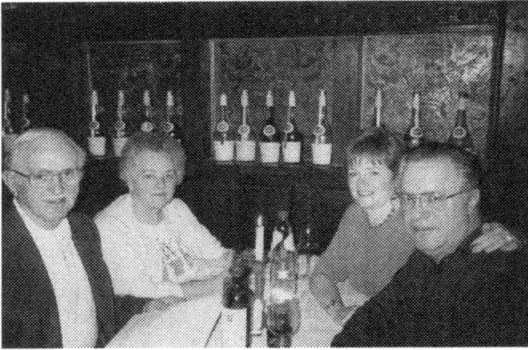

Bob sat on my bed and asked me to try a bite of a dessert that he said was terrific. It was a spongy, creamy dessert called tiramisu, he told me.

to help me (and here's where other people have to start filling in the events for me), but she couldn't. She fell on top of me and decided it would be better to call an ambulance. The paramedics came and took me to the hospital soon enough.

And boy did they find some things wrong with me!

First they found some strange spots on my leg that turned out to be shingles. Shingles is a painful rash caused by the same virus as chicken pox, but they're a lot worse, and the pain makes you tired and sometimes depressed.

I was in such bad shape – the pain from the shingles was overwhelming and I had some paralysis in my right leg – that I wasn't eating or drinking much, and didn't want to get out of bed, either. I lost 45 pounds in two months. Combine this with the fact that I was dehydrated, and it seemed best to everyone that I be checked into the hospital.

So in I went for a stay. They insisted I was only suffering from a very bad case of shingles. They sent me to stay in a rehabilitation hospital for a month and after that, they sent me home to be cared for by a home health aide who had seen me in the hospital.

I wasn't feeling or doing much better than I had at the hospital or the rehab. When the aide came to check on me, she told Marie, "This man is no better today than when I saw him in the hospital. You need to get him back to the doctor."

I was taken to the neurology department at UMass and after being made to suffer through four hours of exams and waiting, I got a new diagnosis – autonomic failure. This is when the autonomic system fails to keep your blood pressure high enough to keep you standing and, in my case, even sitting upright. A large part of the problem was that I was dehydrated.

I was admitted to the hospital immediately and was given loads of fluids. As my pressure began to creep back up, I started to regain some strength. I was released back to Fairlawn for more rehab and this time I was able to participate in my therapy.

While I was in the hospital, some funny things happened to me. I was on so many different drugs, and so mixed up, that I started hallucinating.

I remember a few of these incidents vividly.

In one, Marie and I were at some sort of nightclub with a huge swimming pool in the floor. There were a bunch of young women swimming in it, naked. I couldn't see anything really, but I could tell they were having a good time.

The next day I told Marie that she had to take me back to that nightclub. "Where?" she asked.

"The nightclub where the naked girls are swimming," I told her.

You can imagine how she looked at me!

Another of my hallucinations concerned one of the nurses. She was a black woman and had a really nice shape on her. She used to wear these very tight white pants that I liked and I would kid her about them sometimes.

One night, I woke up and found the room dark and I

wasn't sure where I was. Suddenly, this nurse came into my room – naked! And then she got in bed with me! Of course, it was too dark for me to really see much.

"Gee, thanks," I said to her. "But there's nothing I can do. I'm an 80-year-old man."

She got mad and left. I thought she'd gone to another room to meet up with someone else.

The next day, she came to see me. Not remembering if it had been a hallucination or not, I just kept my mouth shut!

The last strange thing I remember is that I was always telling Marie that aliens were coming into my room at night to get me. Well, this one made no sense to any of us until we realized that the cleaning crew that came into my room at night sometimes moved the furniture to clean!

Not everything about my stay was funny. When I was in getting my therapy, the doctors greatly overmedicated me. Michelle and Lynne told me about one day when they came to visit and found me slumped over in a wheelchair, drooling on myself.

They approached the social worker on my case and told her that this wasn't normal for me, that I was being overmedicated. She asked them if they'd ever seen me sick!

Well, 30 minutes later when they were done telling the stories of all the times they'd seen me sick, the social worker believed them and I was taken off one of my medications – neurontin. There are lawsuits now about people who died from this drug, so I'm glad I got off it when I did. That perked me up some.

Even after I was released and went to stay with Michelle and Bob, things were tough. I was so weak and so sick that I stopped eating much at all and spent most of my days in bed. But tiramisu saved me.

My son-in-law, Bob, came up to my room to see me one day that summer. Since I hadn't been eating, everyone was worried about me. Bob sat on my bed and asked me to try a bite of a dessert that he said was terrific. It was a spongy, creamy dessert called tiramisu, he told me. I was in no mood to try anything, but Bob kept asking me to just try a bite. I kept saying no and he kept saying yes until I finally gave in.

I took a bite and everything changed. What a wonderful dessert.

And after that, not only did I start eating, but I started to get out of bed regularly and was quickly on my way to recovery. And it was the tiramisu that did it!

When I finally came out of my state, I found the Red Sox were in the World Series. After so many decades of near misses, heartbreaking losses, and general sports agony, I couldn't believe it. I thought it was a miracle.

"God's given me a winner before I die!" I thought.

Conclusion

As much as I enjoy summers in Massachusetts, I also have a great time in our winter home in Florida. We first moved there after driving in a mobile home to the world's fair in New Orleans in 1984. From there, we went to Grand Island, Florida, to visit my brother Edward and his wife Louise. We liked it so much that we stayed.

Now we usually head down in early October after having spent the late spring and summer in the north. We fly to Florida and our son in law, John, drives our van back to Florida. He often gets to our home before we do – and he has to drive from Massachusetts!

Life in Florida is leisurely and great, nowhere near as hectic as it is in Massachusetts. We chum around with our neighbors, go out to eat and to the movies, have fun. I take photos. Marie plays bingo about six times a week and we play Mexican dominoes with our neighbors and Marie's brother, who also lives in the area.

Sometimes I go to Marie's brother's house to take photographs of wood ducks. It's quiet there and between photos sometimes I'll take a nap. Other times we head over to

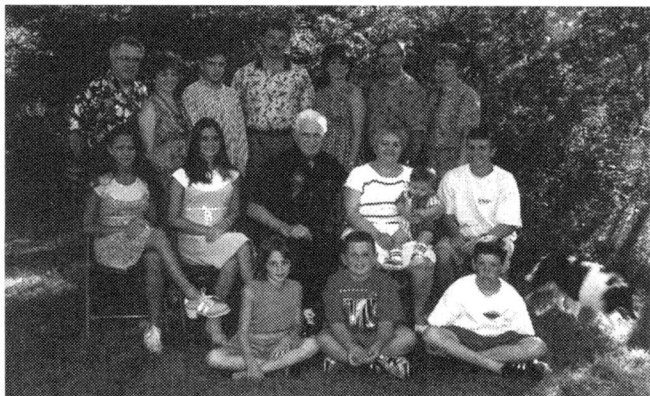

St. Augustine, where there's a rookery and alligator farm. Birds have taken over the place because the raccoons left – they're afraid of the gators. Between the gators and the birds, it makes for some great photos.

We used to go bowling, but my doctors aren't sure I'll be able to go anymore thanks to an aneurysm I have in my stomach. The doctors are afraid that if I lift anything too heavy – more than 25 pounds – it could burst and that would be it for me. These restrictions are too bad because I used to go to the Y three days a week and lift 93 pounds five times to stay in shape. Not anymore, though. At least not for a little while. I'll get back to it.

The first place we lived in Florida was called Southern Palms. In the time we lived there we made some wonderful friends. Chief among them are Earl and Joan Grant, who directed entertainment for Southern Palms.

After doing that work, they took on a bigger challenge: fighting cancer. Joan and Earl have been battling cancer since Earl was diagnosed with colon cancer in the middle 90s. In that time they've built a wonderful organization, the Cancer Society of Leesburg. Every year they host a wonderful survivors dinner in which those of us who have survived cancer get together to eat, joke, hug, and discuss our good luck.

Of course we've lost some people over the years, and that's been sad, but most of us come back for the dinner each year and we have some survivors who have made it 35 years or more. I'm on year 30 myself.

For years my friends have asked me, "when are you going to slow down?" I've never felt like I wanted to and I still don't. I thought maybe I was going to slow down in my 40s, but it didn't happen. I don't remember my 50s well due to my illnesses; that's when it seemed like my world was coming apart. Back then I didn't think I'd even get to 65.

But I celebrated my 70th birthday at a big party with my children and grandchildren and in the summer of 2005 celebrated my 81st birthday surrounded by friends and family.

There were many years when I never thought I'd see 80. Now I keep holding on, looking forward to every day, to new things. I can't wait to spend more time with my great-grandchildren. I hope to see them grow and to give them memories of Marie and me that they can grow up with, the same way I grew up comforted and guided by memories of and experiences with my family.

The biggest thing I'm looking forward to comes in the summer of 2006: my 60th wedding anniversary with Marie. More than anything else, I'm looking forward to seeing that day.

In my life I've seen the world, served in a war, fought and conquered numerous illnesses. What I've learned, though, is that nothing is more important than laughter, love, and family. I've been graced with tremendous amounts of them and have lived a wonderful life because of it.

I hope that in reading my story you've laughed a bit and found some ideas about how to live your life. If I've helped you, even a little, then I've done my job. I hope that you've had a chance to think about your life, about the ways in which you've been challenged and blessed, and how you can live the life you want.

Postscript

In November 2005, just as I was coming to the end of this book, the latest chapter in my health struggles was opened when my doctors in Florida found a spot in my bladder. Of course this usually means cancer.

I'm not a stranger to cancer, of course, but I'm not a stranger to fighting it either. So, once again, I'll call on my sense of humor, my friends, my family, and the love that surrounds me.

Here I go again!

The message on my answering machine from my father said "Michelle, I have some very, very, very, very bad news. Please call me." His voice broke as he spoke the words. After 31 years my dad finally heard the words that he had expected so many times before, "Chick, you don't have long to live. Go up north and be with your family. Get there next week," Dr. Fernandez had told him.

Dad had lost 20 pounds since returning to Florida on October 19, 2005, and it was only December 15th. Dr. Fernandez sent Dad for a CAT scan and the results were that cancer had spread throughout his body: lesions were found on his lungs, liver, kidneys, and the lymph nodes in his groin were enlarged. He and my mom flew back up to my home in Worcester on Tuesday, December 20th.

Dad was happy to be with all of us. He kept saying that he was having a "living wake". He wanted to see his family, hug them, tell them that he loved them and he was able to do it. He passed away on December 23rd. He kept telling us "Goodnight." He was obviously very tired and ready to move on to his next adventure.

What kept this wonderful man going for the past 31 years, since his first cancer? I believe it was always having a future to look forward to. There was always a trip to take, a child to see grow up, a birthday to reach. Even as he spoke of his death he was planning to have his family live out his last dreams. There will be an exhibit of the flower photos that he took during the summer of 2005 at the Italian American Cultural Center in **Worcester** in June 2006. He printed all the photos before he came north. The only thing he left undone was his 60th anniversary with my mom. I know that it makes him mad that it is left to be celebrated without him.

Yet Chick's message is to keep looking ahead. When things get tough, tell a joke or flirt or do something to bring a smile to your face. His most important message was that he loved his family and friends and everyone that he came in contact with.

— Michelle Currie
Chick's eldest daughter
Worcester, MA.
January 2006

About Sam Costello

Sam Costello is a writer living in Providence, RI. His non-fiction has appeared in such diverse publications as CNN.com and *Rue Morgue*, *PC World* and *Bitch*. His short comics have appeared in a number of anthologies and his fiction has been published in *Punk Planet*.

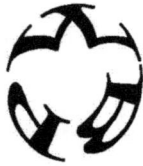

Wandering Brothers Publishing, CO

ISBN 0-9724917-7-5
copyright 2006 Conrad Boilard

cover photo by Harold T. Ahern, FPSA, PPSA
of Belchertown, MA, taken while on a "Photo Safari"
to a wild animal farm in Colorado

www.ingramcontent.com/pod-product-compliance
Lightning Source LLC
Chambersburg PA
CBHW030021290326
41934CB00005B/438